HOOP FUN FOR E

AN INSTRUCTOR'S COMPLETE DEVELOPMENTAL PROGRAM FOR STUDENTS OF ALL AGES

by
GARRY L. SMITH

EDITOR
Frank Alexander

TEXT ARTISTS
Dawn Bates and Holger Jensen

COVER ARTIST
Dawn Bates

CHESTERFIELD COUNTY
Parks and Recreation Department
6801 Wagners Way Road
P. O. Box 40
Chesterfield, VA 23832

Community Recreation

Published by FRONT ROW EXPERIENCE, 540 Discovery Bay Blvd., Byron, CA 94514-9454

500 Books In Print As Of 1993

Copyright © P.E.T.A., Inc. 1993

ISBN 0-915256-35-5

Published

by

FRONT ROW EXPERIENCE
540 Discovery Bay Blvd.
Byron, CA 94514-9454

All rights reserved.
No part of this book may be reproduced
in any form or by any means
without written permission in writing
from the publisher.

ACKNOWLEDGEMENT

I dedicate this book to Larry S. Herrold, Supervisor of Elementary Physical Education for the Baltimore County Public School System in Maryland, and to my four fellow Instructional Specialists for Elementary Physical Education: Ed Lanehart, Sally Nazelrod, Ann Pruett, and Don Williams. For the past number of years we have strived to improve the quality of the elementary physical education program for the tens of thousands of elementary level boys and girls within our vast school system. Through an ongoing process of system based curriculum development and revisions along with the sharing of the elementary physical education curriculum through inservice courses, countywide meetings, area meetings, newsletters, and, most importantly, one on one contacts with fellow colleagues, I feel we have heightened the overall level of the elementary physical education program in Baltimore County. Currently, I strongly feel our elementary physical education program is one of the best within the state of Maryland and, consequently, one of the finest in the nation. It is my only professional hope that we will be able to continue in this positive direction and, somehow, make it through the ever present budget challenges that face my county's school system. In addition, it is my hope that elementary physical education programs across the United States will continue to move in the same positive direction while addressing similar budget challenges. Together, we have an important common-ground mission to accomplish: to help to create a more physically educated child.

ABOUT THE AUTHOR

Garry L. Smith is an Instructional Specialist in Elementary Physical Education in the Baltimore County Public School System, Baltimore County, Maryland. He holds a B.S. degree in Health, Physical Education, & Recreation from Lock Haven State University, Lock Haven, Pennsylvania (1972) and a Master of Education degree in Administration from Western Maryland College, Westminister, Maryland (1978).

He has presented numerous demonstrations/workshops at the elementary and middle school/junior high school levels in county school systems throughout Maryland; as well as at various conventions, conferences, and meetings in the northeast, southeast, and western sections of the country. He has received professional awards at the county, state, and eastern district levels including the Maryland Association of Health, Physical Education, Recreation & Dance Elementary Physical Education Teacher of the Year (1990) and Eastern District Elementary Physical Education Teacher of the Year (1990).

In 1985, Garry founded P.E.T.A. (Physical Education Teaching Accessories), Inc. He has authored two books that are "an instructor's complete developmental program for students of all ages": FUN STUNTS AND TUMBLING STUNTS and PARALLEL BARS. In addition, he has created one hundred and seventy-seven gymnastic charts covering a complete range of beginner and intermediate stunts in nine gymnastic areas: fun (developmental) stunts, tumbling, balance beam, parallel bars, basic jumps, vaulting, horizontal bar, rings, and side horse. To reinforce the skill development in various gymnastic areas, he created five different motivational certificates: Gymnastics, Balance Beam, Parallel Bars, Tumbling, and Vaulting. Also, he has created sixteen hoop charts covering the basic sixteen individual hoop skills.

Garry L. Smith brings twenty one years of experience and expertise in Physical Education together with the talents of professional designers, illustrators, and printers to produce the most unique, attractive, and instructional book for the hoop.

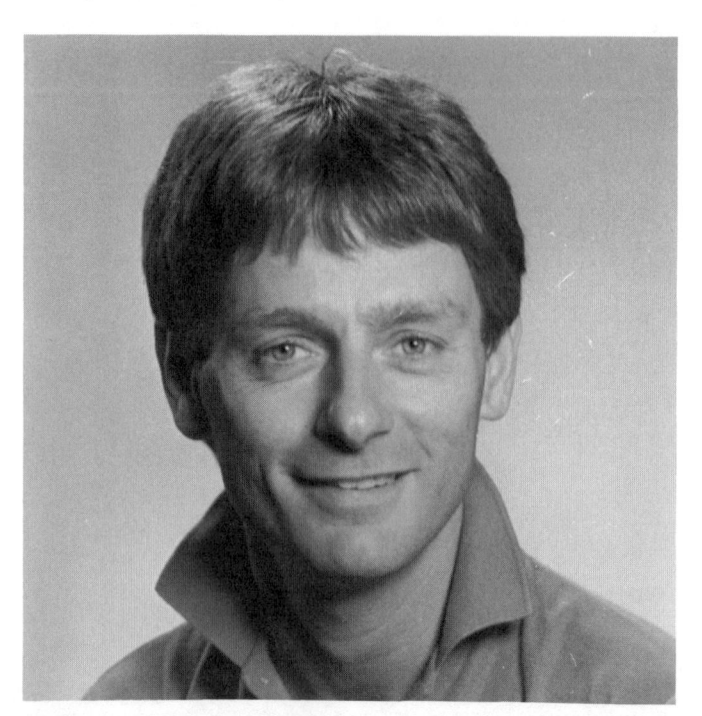

TABLE OF CONTENTS

Preface ---1

Chapter One
SPECIFIC TEACHING SUGGESTIONS AND SAFETY GUIDELINES ----------------3

Chapter Two
THE SIXTEEN BASIC HOOP SKILLS --6

    Spin The Hoop ---6
    Toss And Catch With Right Hand --7
    Toss And Catch With Left Hand ---9
    Backspin ---10
    Hoop Twirl On Waist Forward And Backward ------------------------------11
    Hoop Twirl On Waist Sideward --13
    Hoop Twirl On Neck --14
    Hoop Twirl On Right Wrist Push And Lift -------------------------------15
    Hoop Twirl On Left Wrist Push And Lift--------------------------------16
    Hoop Twirl On Right Wrist Rock Back And Forth -------------------------18
    Hoop Twirl On Left Wrist Rock Back And Forth --------------------------19
    Hoop Exchange On Wrist --20
    Hoop Jumping Pendulum Swings --22
    Hoop Jumping Forward --23
    Hoop Jumping Backward ---24
    Hoop Twirl On Ankle ---26

Chapter Three
ADDITIONAL MANIPULATIVE INDIVIDUAL HOOP SKILLS-----------------------28

Chapter Four
INDIVIDUAL ACTIVITIES WITH THE HOOP IN AN OPEN SPACE ON THE FLOOR --30

Chapter Five
PARTNER ACTIVITIES WITH THE HOOP IN AN OPEN SPACE ON THE FLOOR ----34

Chapter Six
ACTIVE GAMES AND ACTIVE RELAY RACES---------------------------------36

    Knock Away--37
    Hoop Toss---38
    Frisbee Hulabee --40
    Bull's-Eye Frisbee ---41
    Shuffle Ball ---42
    Target Toss --44
    Pass Along Relay ---45
    Spear A Hoop Relay ---46
    Hooper--47
    Hoop Maze --49
    Down And Up Relay --50
    Hoop Roll Relay --51
    Through The Hoop Relay ---52

Bibliography---55

PREFACE

This book has been written to help elementary physical education instructors, elementary level classroom teachers, and other professionals in varying capacities who work closely with children. Also, parents could easily benefit from the information shared within this book. I feel this book is one of, if not the most, comprehensive hoop books available on today's market since most information related to the use of a hoop is included in a general curriculum book. The book is an outgrowth of the sixteen basic hoop charts produced by P.E.T.A., Inc.

It is my hope that the readers will become knowledgeable about the various individual, partner, and group activities/games and perhaps proficient in the ability to perform many of the basic hoop skills in order to be able to share the information with children. The use of a hoop is a fun, exciting, and an inexpensive approach to teaching a variety of individual manipulative skills with numerous opportunities to expand the learning experience through partner, small group, and total class activities.

There are six chapters within this book. Chapter One includes twenty SPECIFIC TEACHING SUGGESTIONS AND SAFETY GUIDELINES. The suggestions and guidelines are offered as ideas to consider prior to organizing and teaching a hoop instructional unit and they are based upon twenty-one years of teaching experience at the elementary level. Use these suggestions and guidelines as a beginning, then add to or delete in order to make your hoop instructional unit meet the ability levels of your students and the needs of your physical education program. Chapter Two covers THE SIXTEEN BASIC HOOP SKILLS beginning with Spin The Top and progressing through fourteen skills and ending with Hoop Twirl On The Ankle. Each skill is broken down into the Starting Position and Performance. Next, a Description outlines the overall skill in brief, verbal sentences. These sentences were designed to be used as teaching cues to assist in the teaching of the various skills. Lastly, each skill includes a list of Additional Teaching Suggestions. Since the approach to teaching each skill is similar, there is overlapping throughout the sixteen hoop skills; however, each skill has Additional Teaching Suggestions specific to the skill being addressed. I apologize for the overlapping but I wanted to cover each skill by itself since most readers will use this book as the initial source for hoop information and the instructional approach will be to learn about and teach one hoop skill at a time. Chapter Three covers eleven ADDITIONAL MANIPULATIVE INDIVIDUAL HOOP SKILLS. After successfully teaching the sixteen Basic Hoop Skills, selected ADDITIONAL MANIPULATIVE INDIVIDUAL HOOP SKILLS can be supplemented into the total instructional hoop unit based upon the success level of individual students and/or the total group of students. Chapter Four addresses fifteen INDIVIDUAL ACTIVITIES WITH THE HOOP IN AN OPEN SPACE ON THE FLOOR. The activities range from the performance of locomotor movements in and around the hoop to the use of the hoop as an instructional tool to reinforce throwing and catching skills. In addition, activities are included to reinforce the teaching of basic math concepts and word recognition skills along with an activity to modify the teaching of the dance called the Hokey Pokey. Chapter Five covers six PARTNER ACTIVITIES WITH THE HOOP IN AN OPEN SPACE ON THE FLOOR. Some of the activities are similar to the activities within Chapter Four with modifications made to allow the activities to be performed in partner groups. Also, different activities are included to reinforce throwing, catching, and kicking skills. Chapter Six explains fourteen ACTIVE GAMES AND ACTIVE RELAY RACES. An overview is included for each game sharing information about the organization of the game, equipment needed to play the game, rules of the game, etc. After each overview is a list of Additional Teaching Suggestions. Important tips are shared to help make the game more successful and fun for the students with an emphasis placed on cooperation, sportsmanship, the important role of appropriate values displayed within the game, etc. Following Chapter Six is a comprehensive Bibliography listing additional sources containing hoop related information. I sincerely hope you find this book to be a valuable resource to you as you continue to provide the best possible physical education program and/or learning experiences for the young people within your teaching environment. Best wishes!

Chapter One
SPECIFIC TEACHING SUGGESTIONS AND SAFETY GUIDELINES

1) Always make certain you have more than enough equipment (hoops) for the students so they realize there will be equipment (hoops) not being used. In so doing, the students will not rush to get equipment (hoops).

2) Find a quick and efficient way to disperse the hoops to the students. Do not place the hoops in one pile and have the students line up to get them. Instead, place the hoops individually around the perimeter of the activity area or throughout the activity area. Consider placing large traffic cones around the perimeter of the activity area with three to five hoops around each cone.

3) Discuss proper use and care of the hoop. Make every student be responsible for the proper use and care of his/her hoop. In particular, discuss what happens to a hoop if someone uses it incorrectly and it no longer remains in a circular shape. If bent, the hoop can no longer be used as a hoop.

4) Make certain the students understand and respect personal space and the personal space of others.

5) Make certain you have and use designated boundaries especially if your teaching station is a gymnasium, activity room, multipurpose room, cafetorium, etc., because there has to be sufficient space between the activity area and the four walls or other obstacles. Do not make the walls or obstacles the designated boundaries.

6) Talk about safety while using the hoop. Address such concerns as throwing the hoop under control; keeping the hoop close to one's self and within one's personal space unless one is asked to perform a specific movement while using the hoop; moving safely and carefully in, out, around, under, over, through, etc., the hoop in a way that the hoop does not touch a fellow classmate.

7) Personally, I do not recommend "airborne" locomotor movements while moving over one side of the hoop or over the whole hoop, namely, jumping, hopping and leaping. If done incorrectly or unsuccessfully, the weight of the student coming down on the hoop sometimes forces the hoop to slide across the ground surface. This could result in an unnecessary injury to the student.

8) Always give the students sufficient practice time to attempt to learn "newly" taught or "previously" taught hoop skills. During the practice time, move throughout the group of students to further individualize the instruction by offering words of assistance, correction, encouragement, and praise.

9) If appropriate, give the students a brief "open practice" time prior to beginning the instructional segment of the lesson. A lot of learning takes place through individual exploration time.

10) Combine teacher demonstrations with student demonstrations. Student demonstrations allow opportunities to informally assess student accomplishments and they provide opportunities to help students develop positive self concepts.

11) Always include a demonstration as part of the teaching process. Since most learners are visual learners, the "total picture" is vital to the learning process.

12) Use charts, commercial or homemade, to reinforce the learning experience. The basic sixteen hoop charts developed by my company, P.E.T.A., Inc., are excellent to use to reinforce the learning process. Also, the use of charts allows for a station approach to learning.

13) Always offer words of praise and encouragement to all students regardless of their specific ability levels assuming the students were on task and giving their best effort.

14) Always make student praise effective and part of the total learning process. Instead of using one and two word positive feedback such as "Great" or "Nice Job," clarify the meaning of the initial one or two words by emphasizing the reasoning of the praise. For example, "Johnny, Super! You really are being successful because you are making your arm move up and down" (Hoop Twirl On The Wrist) or "Susan, you're terrific! I like the way you are controlling the release of your hoop" (Backspin). Make the praise short and to the point. Also, say it loud enough for all students to hear. This way, individual praise can be reinforcement for proper technique to all the students.

15) If possible, ask the classroom teacher to observe or take an active instructional role at various points throughout the hoop skills and activities unit. This way, the classroom teacher will be able to do follow-up teaching and reinforcement of learning during supervised play.

16) Use cooperative teaching techniques to enhance the learning experiences. For example, include reciprocal teaching opportunities within the lessons to give students time to assist each other with the learning process or explain pair/share and include this technique within the instructional segment of the lesson or within the lesson summary. Always strive for a high activity level within all phases of the teaching process.

17) Integrate educational values into the hoop skills and activities unit by highlighting such values as honesty, courtesy, responsibility, respect for the rights of others, human worth and dignity, sportsmanship, etc., at meaningful and appropriate times.

18) Integrate other curriculum areas into the lesson through the use of word cards to reinforce directional concepts with related movements or use a portable chalkboard, large piece of paper, etc., to write a math problem and have the students record the answer by placing the answer on a card in a hoop. (Refer to Chapter Four, INDIVIDUAL ACTIVITIES WITH THE HOOP IN AN OPEN SPACE ON THE FLOOR, or Chapter Five, PARTNER ACTIVITIES WITH THE HOOP IN AN OPEN SPACE ON THE FLOOR, for further clarification.)

19) Parallel your hoop unit with a totally different unit to allow for varied learning experiences. Examples are hoop skills and activities combined with one of the following instructional units: rhythms and dance, striking skills and activities, ball skills progression, individual fitness and exercise, distance jogging, etc. According to the needs of your students, divide the total class time into two sections. Then, teach skills and activities specific to one of the units within each section.

20) After the completion of your hoop skills and activities unit, practice specific skills in future lessons as the warm-up session. For example, use Hoop Jump Forward and Hoop Jump Backward as the aerobic phase of warm-up sessions or have the students continue to practice Hoop Twirl On Waist: Forward And Backward and Hoop Twirl On Waist: Sideward in attempts to increase their times for the Hoop Time Clubs.

Chapter Two
THE SIXTEEN BASIC HOOP SKILLS

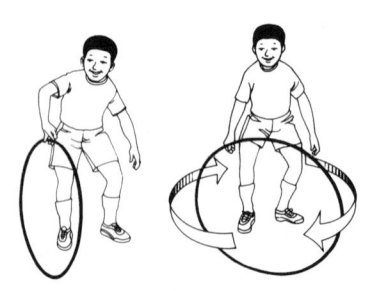

SPIN THE HOOP

STARTING POSITION
Stand in a relaxed position. Hold the hoop in a horizontal position in front of the body. The hand is twisted in preparation to spin the hoop.

PERFORMANCE
Untwist the wrist and let go of the spinning hoop. Step back from the spinning hoop.

DESCRIPTION
Hold the hoop and twist the wrist.
Untwist the wrist.
Let go of the hoop and step back.
Watch the hoop spin like a top.

ADDITIONAL TEACHING SUGGESTIONS

1) Demonstrate and discuss the skill. Break the skills down into its component parts.

2) Introduce the skill in a whole/part and part/whole teaching technique progression.

3) Relate the skill "Spin The Hoop" to "Spin The Top". Use a top to demonstrate "Spin The Top".

4) Discuss words with the same meaning as spin: turn, twirl, circle, rotate, etc.

5) Discuss the difference between the two non-locomotor movements: twist and turn (spin).

6) Stress the importance of having one's personal space and staying within the personal space.

7) Practice the twisting action of the wrist without the hoop then transfer the learning experience to the use of the hoop.

8) Give ample practice time.

9) Move throughout the group during the practice sessions to individualize the instruction. Praise and encourage all students regardless of their ability levels.

10) Use students who are successful with the skill to assist those who need additional assistance. Stress cooperation, human worth and dignity, and compassion.

11) Challenge students to travel around the spinning hoop while performing a variety of locomotor movements: walk, march, jog, run, hop, jump, gallop, skip, etc.

12) Have the students travel in both directions around the spinning hoop; clockwise and counterclockwise. Make certain the students understand the meaning of the terms.

13) Have all students begin to spin the hoops at the same time to see which hoop spins for the longest period of time. Ask students to point to the hoop that spins the longest.

14) Prior to having the students begin to spin the hoops in #13 above, take advantage of the teaching situation to stress the value: honesty. Each student must begin the spin at the same time and once the hoop is released, it cannot be touched.

15) Give the students opportunities to demonstrate the skill. Have classmates clap for the demonstrators.

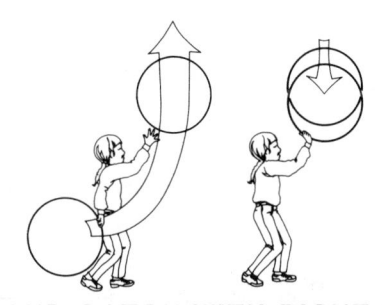

TOSS AND CATCH WITH RIGHT HAND

STARTING POSITION
Stand in a relaxed position. Hold the hoop (overhand grip) in the right hand on the right side of the body.

PERFORMANCE
Lift and toss the hoop directly overhead. Watch the hoop travel upward then downward. Catch the hoop at a safe distance in front of the forehead. The thumb and fingers wrap around the hoop.

DESCRIPTION
Hold the hoop with the right hand.
Lift and toss the hoop.
Watch the hoop travel upward then downward.
Catch the hoop with the right hand.

ADDITIONAL TEACHING SUGGESTIONS

1) Demonstrate and discuss the skill. Break the skill down into its component parts.

2) Introduce the skill in a whole/part and part/whole teaching technique progression.

3) Stress the importance of having one's personal space and staying within the personal space.

4) Make certain all tosses are under control. Continually remind the students to toss the hoop directly overhead so each student stays in his/her personal space.

5) Emphasize proper and safe catching skills: track the path of the hoop then reach and grasp the hoop a safe distance in front of the forehead by wrapping the thumb and fingers around the hoop.

6) Give ample practice time.

7) Move throughout the group during the practice sessions to individualize the instruction. Praise and encourage all students regardless of their ability levels.

8) Use students who are successful with the skill to assist those students who need additional assistance. Stress cooperation, human worth and dignity, and compassion.

9) Toss the hoop from hand to hand.

10) Challenge each student to toss the hoop, clap hands one time, and catch the hoop. If successful, have the student add a second clap. Continue to add a clap with each successful catch.

11) Challenge each student to toss the hoop, touch a body part, and catch the hoop. Have the student touch a different body part each time.

12) Challenge each student to toss the hoop, touch a body part, and catch the hoop. If successful, have the student touch the same body part then touch a different body part and catch the hoop. Continue to add a different body part with each successful catch.

13) Challenge each student to toss, turn around, and catch the hoop. If successful, turn in the other direction. Discuss clockwise and counterclockwise.

14) Give the students opportunities to demonstrate the skill. Have classmates clap for the demonstrators.

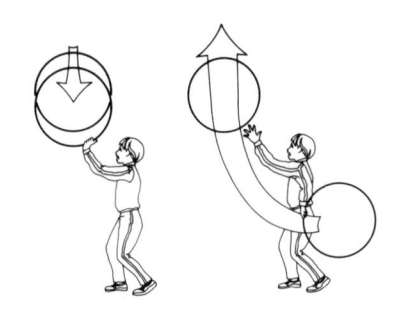

TOSS AND CATCH WITH LEFT HAND

STARTING POSITION
Stand in a relaxed position. Hold the hoop (overhand grip) in the left hand on the left side of the body.

PERFORMANCE
Lift and toss the hoop directly overhead. Watch the hoop travel upward then downward. Catch the hoop at a safe distance in front of the forehead. The thumb and fingers wrap around the hoop.

DESCRIPTION
Hold the hoop with the left hand.
Lift and toss the hoop.
Watch the hoop travel upward then downward.
Catch the hoop with the left hand.

ADDITIONAL TEACHING SUGGESTIONS

1) Demonstrate and discuss the skill. Break the skill down into its component parts.

2) Introduce the skill in a whole/part and part/whole teaching technique progression.

3) Stress the importance of having one's personal space and staying within the personal space.

4) Make certain all tosses are under control. Continually remind the students to toss the hoop directly overhead so each student stays in his/her personal space.

5) Emphasize proper and safe catching skills: track the path of the hoop then reach and grasp the hoop a safe distance in front of the forehead by wrapping the thumb and fingers around the hoop.

6) Give ample practice time.

7) Move throughout the group during the practice sessions to individualize the instruction. Praise and encourage all students regardless of their ability levels.

8) Use students who are successful with the skill to assist those students who need additional assistance. Stress cooperation, human worth and dignity and compassion.

9) Toss the hoop from hand to hand.

10) Challenge each student to toss the hoop, clap hands one time, and catch the hoop. If successful, have the student add a second clap. Continue to add a clap with each successful catch.

11) Challenge each student to toss the hoop, touch a body part, and catch the hoop. Have the student touch a different body part each time.

12) Challenge each student to toss the hoop, touch a body part, and catch the hoop. If successful, have the student touch the same body part then touch a different body part and catch the hoop. Continue to add a different body part with each successful catch.

13) Challenge each student to toss, turn around, and catch the hoop. If successful, turn in the other direction. Discuss clockwise and counterclockwise.

14) Give the students opportunities to demonstrate the skill. Have classmates clap for the demonstrators.

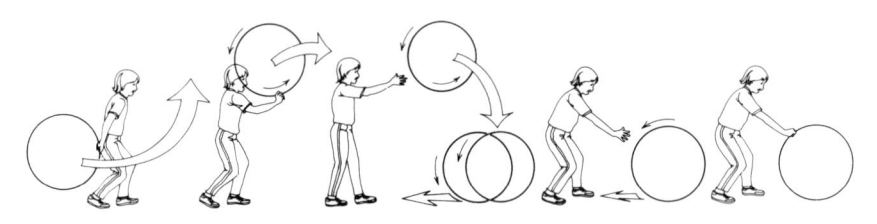

BACKSPIN

STARTING POSITION
Stand in a relaxed position. Hold the hoop in the right or left hand on the same side of the body.

PERFORMANCE
Swing the hoop forward, upward, and backward. Let go of the hoop by snapping the wrist and hand backward and downward. Send the hoop forward with a backward spin. Have the student catch the hoop when it returns to him/her.

DESCRIPTION
Hold the hoop with right or left hand.
Swing the hoop forward, upward, and backward.
Snap the wrist and let go of the hoop.
Watch the hoop travel forward then backward.
Catch the rolling hoop.

ADDITIONAL TEACHING SUGGESTIONS

1) Demonstrate and discuss the skill. Break the skill down into its component parts.

2) Introduce the skill in a whole/part and part/whole teaching technique progression.

3) Stress the importance of having one's personal space and staying within the personal space.

4) Discuss the meaning of "backspin" and make certain the students understand the process.

5) Give ample practice time.

6) Move throughout the group during the practice sessions to individualize the instruction. Praise and encourage all students regardless of their ability levels.

7) Give individualized assistance, if necessary. Stand behind the student and hold the student's hand which is gripping the hoop. Take the student's hand through the proper movements a few times before allowing the hoop to be released. Then, encourage the student to practice.

8) Use students who are successful with the skill to assist those students who need additional assistance. Stress cooperation, human worth and dignity, and compassion.

9) Challenge the students to release the hoop with varying intensities in an attempt to have the hoop travel a specific distance forward before starting to return.

10) Once the student has mastered the skill with the dominate hand, encourage the student to attempt to practice the skill with the opposite hand.

11) If the student can perform the skill with each hand, challenge the student to alternate the skill from right hand to left hand then left hand to right hand. Continue the process.

12) Give the students opportunities to demonstrate the skill. Have classmates clap for the demonstrators.

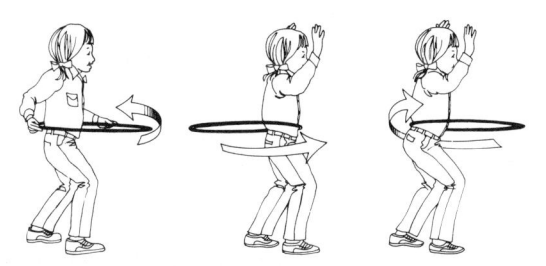

**HOOP TWIRL ON WAIST
FORWARD AND BACKWARD**

STARTING POSITION
Stand in a relaxed position with one foot in front of the other foot. The knees are bent and the hands are in overhand grip positions on the sides of the hoop. The inside of the hoop is touching the lower back.

PERFORMANCE
Toss the hoop in a circular direction around the waist and immediately let go. By keeping the knees bent and the body in an upright, relaxed position, rock the hips in continuous forward and backward movements to allow the hoop to twirl around the waist.

DESCRIPTION
Hold the hoop at the waist.
Toss the hoop around the waist.
Let go of the hoop.

Rock the hips forward and backward.
Keep the knees bent and the body relaxed.
Feel the hoop twirl around the waist.

ADDITIONAL TEACHING SUGGESTIONS

1) Demonstrate and discuss the skill. Break the skill down into its component parts.

2) Introduce the skill in a whole/part and part/whole teaching technique progression.

3) Stress the importance of having one's personal space and staying within the personal space.

4) Have the students practice the forward and backward rocking movements without the hoop before using the hoop.

5) Make certain the students keep their feet in the proper position, one foot in front of the other foot, during all phases of the skill.

6) Tell the students to lift the hands immediately after releasing the hoop so the hands do not interfere with the twirling movement of the hoop.

7) Discuss the importance of keeping the shoulders and head stationary during the rocking movements.

8) Give ample practice time.

9) Move throughout the group during the practice sessions to individualize the instruction. Praise and encourage all students regardless of their ability levels.

10) Use students who are successful with the skill to assist those students who need additional assistance. Stress cooperation, human worth and dignity, and compassion.

11) Create a Hoop Time Club wall display and divide the display into time allotments: 15 Seconds, 30 Seconds, 1 Minute, 2 Minutes, 3 Minutes, etc. List the names of the students beginning with 15 Seconds who can Hoop Twirl On The Waist for a specific period of time. Give each student, who at least makes the 15 Seconds time allotment, a "special" certificate. Assuming one's personal best was given, consider a "special effort" certificate for the student who did not reach the 15 Seconds time period.

12) Give the students opportunities to demonstrate the skill. Have classmates clap for the demonstrators.

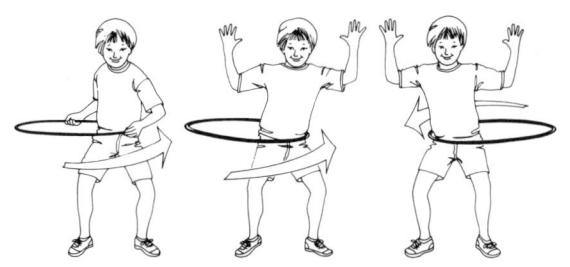

HOOP TWIRL ON WAIST
SIDEWARD

STARTING POSITION
Stand in a relaxed position with the feet slightly greater than shoulder width apart. The knees are bent and the hands are in overhand grip positions on the sides of the hoop. The inside of the hoop is touching the lower back.

PERFORMANCE
Toss the hoop in a circular direction around the waist and immediately let go. By keeping the knees bent and the body in an upright, relaxed position, rock the hips in continuous side to side movements to allow the hoop to twirl around the waist.

DESCRIPTION
Hold the hoop at the waist.
Toss the hoop around the waist.
Let go of the hoop.
Rock the hips side to side.
Keep the knees bent and the body relaxed.
Feel the hoop twirl around the waist.

ADDITIONAL TEACHING SUGGESTIONS

1) Demonstrate and discuss the skill. Break the skill down into its component parts.

2) Introduce the skill in a whole/part and part/whole teaching technique progression.

3) Stress the importance of having one's personal space and staying within the personal space.

4) Have students practice the side to side rocking movements without the hoop before using the hoop.

5) Make certain the students keep their feet in the proper position, slightly greater than shoulder width apart, during all phases of the skill.

6) Tell the students to lift the hands immediately after releasing the hoop so the hands do not interfere with the twirling movement of the hoop.

7) Discuss the importance of keeping the shoulders and the head stationary during the rocking movements.

8) Give ample practice time.

9) Move throughout the group during the practice sessions to individualize the instruction. Praise and encourage all students regardless of their ability levels.

10) Use students who are successful with the skill to assist those students who need additional assistance. Stress cooperation, human worth and dignity, and compassion.

11) Create a Hoop Time Club wall display and divide the display into the following time allotments: 15 Seconds, 30 Seconds, 1 Minute, 2 Minutes, 3 Minutes, etc. List the names of the students beginning with 15 Seconds who can Hoop Twirl On The Waist for a specific period of time. Give each student, who at least makes the 15 Seconds time allotment, a "special" certificate. Assuming one's personal best was given, consider a "special effort" certificate for the students who do not reach the 15 Seconds time period.

12) Give the students opportunities to demonstrate the skill. Have classmates clap for the demonstrators.

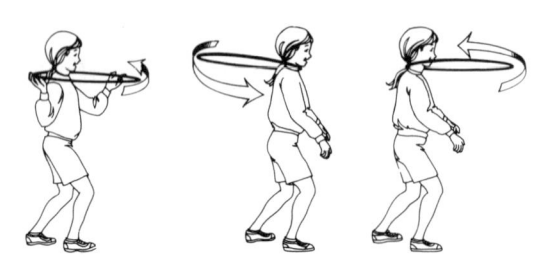

HOOP TWIRL ON NECK

STARTING POSITION
Stand in a relaxed position with one foot in front of the other foot. The knees are bent and the hands are in overhand grip positions on the sides of the hoop. The inside of the hoop is touching the back of the neck.

PERFORMANCE
Toss the hoop in a circular direction around the neck and immediately let go. By keeping the knees bent and the body in an upright, relaxed position, rock the mid and upper body in continuous forward and backward movements to allow the hoop to twirl around the neck.

DESCRIPTION
Hold the hoop at the neck.
Toss the hoop around the neck.
Let go of the hoop.
Rock the mid and upper body forward and backward.
Keep the knees bent and the body relaxed.
Feel the hoop twirl around the neck.

ADDITIONAL TEACHING SUGGESTIONS

1) Demonstrate and discuss the skill. Break the skill down into its component parts.

2) Introduce the skill in a whole/part and part/whole teaching technique progression.

3) Stress the importance of having one's personal space and staying with the personal space.

4) Have the students practice the forward and backward rocking movements without the hoop before using the hoop.

5) Make certain the students keep their feet in the proper position, one foot in front of the other foot, during all phases of the skill.

6) Tell the students to lower their hands immediately after releasing the hoop so the hands do not interfere with the twirling movement of the hoop.

7) Discuss the need to rock the mid and upper body forward and backward. The body below the waist stays in a relaxed, stationary position.

8) Limit the practice/performance time because the twirling movement can become a little uncomfortable to the neck.

9) Move throughout the group during the practice sessions to individualize the instruction. Praise and encourage all students regardless of their ability levels.

10) Use students who are successful with the skill to assist those students who need additional assistance. Stress cooperation, human worth and dignity, and compassion.

11) Give the students opportunities to demonstrate the skill. Have classmates clap for the demonstrators.

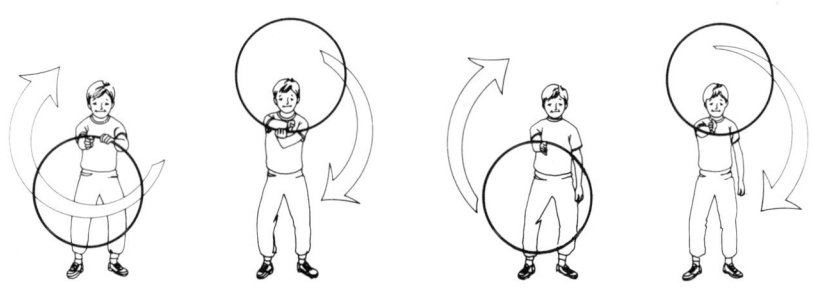

**HOOP TWIRL ON RIGHT WRIST
PUSH AND LIFT**

STARTING POSITION
Stand in a relaxed position with the knees slightly bent and the feet approximately shoulder width apart. The right arm is extended forward with the hoop resting on the inside of the wrist. Use the overhand grip to hold the hoop with the left hand close to the right wrist.

PERFORMANCE
Push the hoop downward then upward to begin the circular movement of the hoop around the right wrist. Simultaneously, lift the right arm. At the height of the circular pathway of the hoop, release the grip. Immediately lower the extended arm to allow the hoop to begin its downward circular movement. Continue the circular movement of the hoop by lifting the arm when the hoop reaches it lowest point. Repeat the downward and upward movement of the arm to allow the hoop to twirl around the right wrist.

DESCRIPTION
Balance the hoop on the right wrist.
Hold the hoop with the left hand (overhand grip).
Push the hoop downward then upward with the left hand.
Lift the right arm.
Release the grip and lower the arm to allow the hoop to twirl around the wrist.
Repeat the arm movements to continue the hoop twirl.

ADDITIONAL TEACHING SUGGESTIONS

1) Demonstrate and discuss the skill. Break the skill down into its component parts.

2) Introduce the skill in a whole/part and part/whole teaching technique progression.

3) Stress the importance of having one's personal space and staying within the personal space.

4) Explain the need to use the overhand grip with the left hand.

5) Discuss the downward then upward push with the left hand to begin the circular movement of the hoop around the right waist.

6) Explain the twirling movement of the hoop around the wrist resulting from the upward and downward movement of the arm.

7) Stress the need to keep the arm extended in front of the body without allowing the arm to rise above shoulder level because a lifted arm allows the hoop to work its way toward the body with eventual hoop to body contact.

8) Make certain the students keep their feet in the proper position, slightly greater than shoulder width apart, during all phases of the skill.

9) Give ample practice time.

10) Give individualized assistance by gently grasping the student's right hand and guiding the hand through all phases of the skill. In the beginning, give the appropriate instructions to have the student push the hoop to perform the downward then upward circular movement of the hoop around the wrist. Release the hand once the student has the proper upward and downward arm movement to permit the hoop to twirl around the wrist. Repeat the process, if necessary.

11) Use students who are successful with the skill to assist those students who need additional assistance. Stress cooperation, human worth and dignity, and compassion.

12) Give the students opportunities to demonstrate the skill. Have classmates clap for the demonstrators.

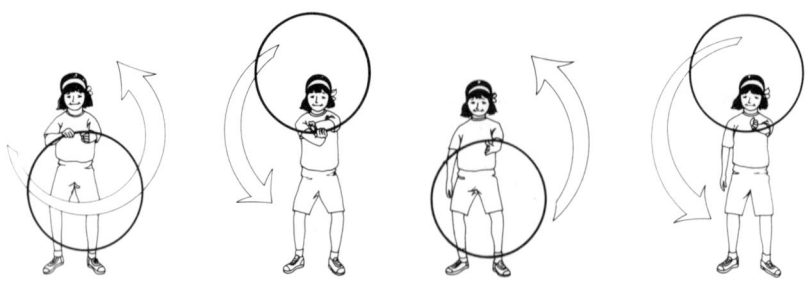

**HOOP TWIRL ON LEFT WRIST
PUSH AND LIFT**

STARTING POSITION
Stand in a relaxed position with the knees slightly bent and the feet approximately shoulder width apart. The left arm is extended forward with the hoop resting on the inside of the wrist. Use the overhand grip to hold the hoop with the right hand close to the left wrist.

PERFORMANCE

Push the hoop downward then upward to begin the circular movement of the hoop around the left wrist. Simultaneously, lift the left arm. At the height of the circular pathway of the hoop, release the grip. Immediately lower the extended arm to allow the hoop to begin its downward circular movement. Continue the circular movement of the hoop by lifting the arm when the hoop reaches its lowest point. Repeat the downward and upward movement of the arm to allow the hoop to twirl around the left wrist.

DESCRIPTION

Balance the hoop on the left wrist.
Hold the hoop with the right hand (overhand grip).
Push the hoop downward then upward with the right hand.
Lift the left arm.
Release the grip and lower the arm to allow the hoop to twirl around the wrist.
Repeat the arm movements to continue the arm twirl.

ADDITIONAL TEACHING SUGGESTIONS

1) Demonstrate and discuss the skill. Break the skill down into its component parts.

2) Introduce the skill in a whole/part and part/whole teaching technique progression.

3) Stress the importance of having one's personal space and staying within the personal space.

4) Explain the need to use the overhand grip with the right hand.

5) Discuss the downward then upward push with the right hand to begin the circular movement of the hoop around the left wrist.

6) Explain the twirling movement of the hoop around the wrist resulting from the upward and downward movement of the arm.

7) Stress the need to keep the arm extended in front of the body without allowing the arm to rise above shoulder level because a lifted arm allows the hoop to work its way toward the body with eventual hoop to body contact.

8) Make certain the students keep their feet in the proper position, slightly greater than shoulder width apart, during all phases of the skill.

9) Give ample practice time.

10) Give individualized assistance by gently grasping the student's left hand and guiding the hand through all phases of the skill. In the beginning, give the appropriate instructions to have the student push the hoop to perform the downward then upward circular movement of the hoop around the wrist. Release the hand once the student has the proper upward and downward arm movement to permit the hoop to twirl around the wrist. Repeat the process, if necessary.

11) Use students who are successful with the skill to assist those students who need additional assistance. Stress cooperation, human worth and dignity, and compassion.

12) Give the students opportunities to demonstrate the skill. Have classmates clap for the demonstrators.

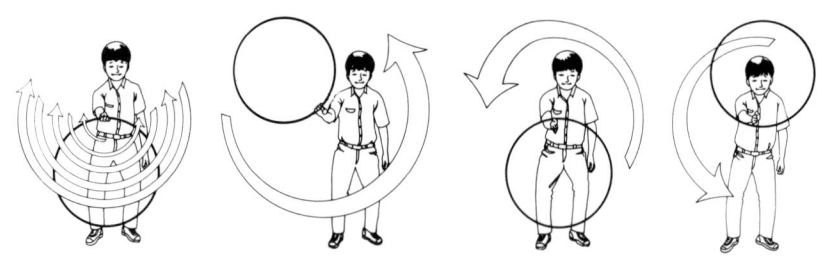

**HOOP TWIRL ON RIGHT WRIST
ROCK BACK AND FORTH**

STARTING POSITION
Stand in a relaxed position with the knees slightly bent and the feet approximately shoulder width apart. The hoop is held in the palm of the right hand with the fingers open and the thumb on top of the hoop.

PERFORMANCE
Lift the hoop by rocking the hoop back and forth beginning on the right side with a gradual increase in height on each swing. At the height of the final swing, grip the hoop and snap the hoop downward and upward. Release the grip by lifting the thumb. At the same time, extend the arm forward at chest level to allow the hoop to continue its upward movement around the wrist. When the hoop reaches its highest point, quickly lower the arm to allow the hoop to begin its downward circular movement. Continue the circular movement of the hoop by lifting the arm when the hoop reaches its lowest point. Repeat the downward and upward movement of the arm to allow the hoop to twirl around the right wrist.

DESCRIPTION
Hold the hoop with the right hand; fingers open and the thumb on top of the hoop.
Rock the hoop from side to side.
Snap the hoop downward, release the grip, and extend the arm forward.
Lower then lift the arm to allow the hoop to twirl around the wrist.
Repeat the arm movements to continue the hoop twirl.

ADDITIONAL TEACHING SUGGESTIONS

1) Demonstrate and discuss the skill. Break the skill down into its component parts.

2) Introduce the skill in a whole/part and part/whole teaching technique progression.

3) Stress the importance of having one's personal space and staying within the personal space.

4) Have the students practice the rocking movement of the hoop with a gradual increase in height on each swing without the eventual release of the hoop.

5) Explain the twirling movement of the hoop around the wrist resulting from the upward and downward movement of the arm.

6) Stress the need to keep the arm extended in front of the body without allowing the arm to rise above shoulder level because a lifted arm allows the hoop to work its way toward the body with eventual hoop to body contact.

7) Discuss the need to snap the hoop downward once the hoop reaches its highest point on the final swing to attain the necessary speed to begin the twirling movement around the wrist.

8) Make certain the students keep their feet in the proper position, slightly greater than shoulder width apart, during all phases of the skill.

9) Give ample practice time.

10) Give individualized assistance by gently grasping the student's right hand and guiding the hand through all phases of the skill. Release the hand once the student has the proper upward and downward arm movement to permit the hoop to twirl around the wrist. Repeat the process, if necessary.

11) Use students who are successful with the skill to assist those students who need additional assistance. Stress cooperation, human worth and dignity, and compassion.

12) Give the students opportunities to demonstrate the skill. Have classmates clap for the demonstrators.

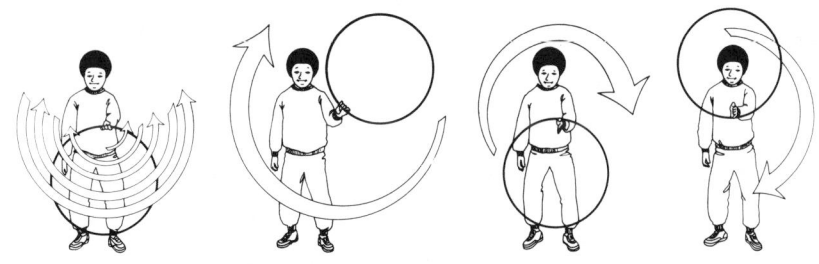

**HOOP TWIRL ON LEFT WRIST
ROCK BACK AND FORTH**

STARTING POSITION
Stand in a relaxed position with the knees slightly bent and the feet approximately shoulder width apart. The hoop is held in the palm of the left hand with the fingers open and the thumb on top of the hoop.

PERFORMANCE
Lift the hoop by rocking the hoop back and forth beginning on the left side with a gradual increase in height on each swing. At the height of the final swing, grip the hoop and snap the hoop downward and upward. Release the grip by lifting the thumb. At the same time, extend the arm forward at the chest level to allow the hoop to continue its upward movement around the wrist. When the hoop reaches its highest point, quickly lower the arm to allow the hoop to begin its downward circular movement. Continue the circular movement of the hoop by lifting the arm when the hoop reaches its lowest point. Repeat the downward and upward movement of the arm to allow the hoop to twirl around the left wrist.

DESCRIPTION
Hold the hoop with the left hand; fingers open and the thumb on top of the hoop.
Rock the hoop from side to side.
Snap the hoop downward, release the grip, and extend the arm forward.
Lower then lift the arm to allow the hoop to twirl around the wrist.
Repeat the arm movements to continue the hoop twirl.

ADDITIONAL TEACHING SUGGESTIONS

1) Demonstrate and discuss the skill. Break the skill down into its component parts.

2) Introduce the skill in a whole/part and part/whole teaching technique progression.

3) Stress the importance of having one's personal space and staying within the personal space.

4) Have the students practice the rocking movement of the hoop with a gradual increase in height on each swing without the eventual release of the hoop.

5) Explain the twirling movement of the hoop around the wrist resulting from the upward and downward movement of the arm.

6) Stress the need to keep the arm extended in front of the body without allowing the arm to rise above shoulder level because a lifted arm allows the hoop to work its way toward the body with eventual hoop to body contact.

7) Discuss the need to snap the hoop downward once the hoop reaches its highest point on the final swing to attain the necessary speed to begin the twirling movement around the wrist.

8) Make certain the students keep their feet in the proper position, slightly greater than shoulder width apart, during all phases of the skill.

9) Give ample practice time.

10) Give individualized assistance by gently grasping the student's left hand and guiding the hand through all phases of the skill. Release the hand once the student has the proper upward and downward arm movement to permit the hoop to twirl around the wrist. Repeat the process, if necessary.

11) Use students who are successful with the skill to assist those students who need additional assistance. Stress cooperation, human worth and dignity, and compassion.

12) Give the students opportunities to demonstrate the skill. Have classmates clap for the demonstrators.

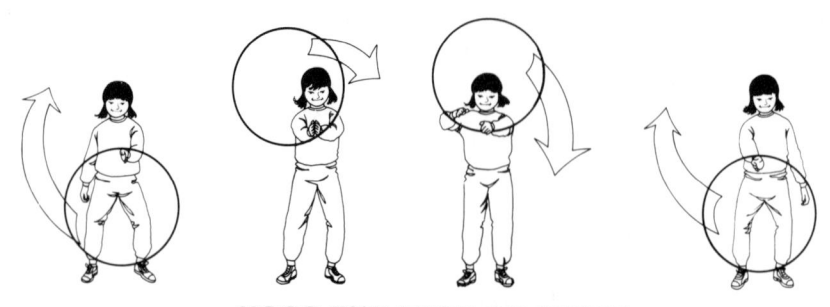

HOOP EXHANGE ON WRIST

STARTING POSITION
Stand in a relaxed position with the knees slightly bent and the feet approximately shoulder width apart. The left arm is extended forward with the hoop at the lowest point of the Hoop Twirl On Left Wrist (refer to page 19 for teaching guidelines).

PERFORMANCE

Continue the Hoop Twirl On Left Wrist by lifting the left arm to allow the hoop to begin its upward circular pathway. At the same time lift the right arm in front of the body. As the hoop begins to reach its highest circular point, extend the right hand into the twirling hoop so the hoop twirls around both wrists. Immediately, pull out the left hand to permit the hoop to twirl around the right wrist. Lower the right arm to allow the hoop to begin its downward circular pathway. At the same time, lower the left arm to place the arm beside the body. Continue the Hoop Exchange On Wrist by repeating the process: lift the right arm, lift then extend the left hand into the twirling hoop as the hoop begins to reach its highest circular point so the hoop twirls around both wrists, pull out the right hand, lower the left arm, and place the right arm beside the body. In order to continue the Hoop Exchange On Wrist, lift the left arm and repeat all steps beginning with the extension of the right hand into the elevated twirling hoop.

DESCRIPTION

Twirl the hoop on the left wrist.
Lift the left arm.
Extend the right hand into the elevated hoop.
Pull out the left hand.
Twirl the hoop on the right wrist.
Lower the right arm.
Repeat the process: lift the right arm.

ADDITIONAL TEACHING SUGGESTIONS

1) Demonstrate and discuss the skill. Break the skill down into its component parts.

2) Introduce the skill in a whole/part and part/whole teaching technique progression.

3) Stress the importance of having one's personal space and staying within the personal space.

4) Make certain the students are successful with Hoop Twirl On Right Wrist and Hoop Twirl On Left Wrist prior to attempting Hoop Exchange On Wrist.

5) Explain and demonstrate the timing of the left or right hand being extended into the twirling hoop as the hoop almost reaches its highest circular point.

6) After the hand is extended into the hoop, make certain the other hand is immediately pulled out to allow the hoop to begin its downward twirl on the inserted hand/wrist.

7) Make certain the students keep their feet in the proper position, slightly greater than shoulder width apart, during all phases of the skill.

8) Give ample practice time.

9) Use students who are successful with the skill to assist those students who need additional assistance. Stress cooperation, human worth and dignity, and compassion.

10) Give the students opportunities to demonstrate the skill. Have classmates clap for the demonstrators.

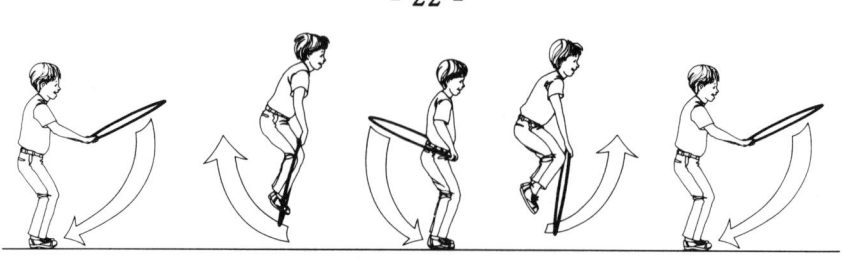

HOOP JUMPING
PENDULUM SWINGS

STARTING POSITION
Begin in a bent leg, relaxed standing position with the feet together. The arms are extended forward with the hands grasping the hoop in front of the waist. The hoop is slightly elevated above the parallel level with the ground surface and the hands are in an overhand grip position while being approximately shoulder width apart on the hoop.

PERFORMANCE
Lower the arms and swing the hoop in a downward direction. As the hoop passes below the level of the knees, jump directly upward to allow the hoop to swing under the feet. After the hoop passes under the feet, begin to swing the hoop upward behind the body. Land in a bent leg, relaxed position on the balls of the feet inside the hoop. The hands are positioned directly in front of the hips and the hoop is slightly elevated above the parallel level with the ground surface. Next, swing the hoop in a downward direction. As the hoop passes below the level of the knees, jump directly upward to allow the hoop to swing under the feet. After the hoop passes under the feet, begin to swing the hoop upward in front of the body. Land in a bent leg, relaxed position on the balls of the feet. The arms are extended forward with the hands grasping the hoop in front of the waist. The hoop is slightly elevated above the parallel level with the ground surface and the hands are in an overhand grip position while being approximately shoulder width apart on the hoop. Repeat the procedure to continue Hoop Jumping Pendulum Swings.

DESCRIPTION
Hold the hoop in front of the body with an overhand grip.
Swing the hoop downward, under, and upward behind the body.
Jump the hoop as it passes under the feet.
Swing the hoop downward, under, and upward in front of the body.
Jump the hoop as it passes under the feet.
Continue to jump using pendulum swings.

ADDITIONAL TEACHING SUGGESTIONS

1) Demonstrate and discuss the skill. Break the skill down into its component parts.

2) Introduce the skill in a whole/part and part/whole teaching technique progression.

3) Stress the importance of having one's personal space and staying within the personal space.

4) Explain a pendulum and how it works.

5) Encourage the students to use the overhand grip.

6) Make certain the students keep their hands approximately shoulder width apart on the hoop.

7) Emphasize the need to keep the chin level and the shoulders back throughout the entire performance of the skill. Allowing the chin to drop and the shoulders to move forward results in loss of balance and the opportunity for the student to fall.

8) Stress the proper landing technique: bend knees, keep chin level, and land on balls of feet.

9) Discuss the movement of the hands and wrists to allow the hoop to swing backward then forward in continuous motion.

10) Challenge the students to continue the pendulum swings and jumps without stopping.

11) Have the students perform different styles of jumping/passing over the hoop: single jump rebound/double jump, hop, gallop, skip, etc.

12) Use students who are successful with the skill to assist those students who need additional assistance. Stress cooperation, human worth and dignity, and compassion.

13) Give the students opportunities to demonstrate the skill. Have classmates clap for the demonstrators.

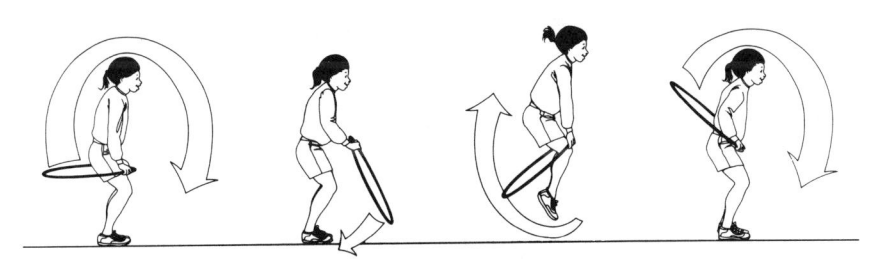

HOOP JUMPING FORWARD

STARTING POSITION
Begin in a bent leg, relaxed standing position inside the hoop with the feet together. The arms are extended downward with the hands grasping the hoop at mid thigh level. The hoop is parallel with the ground surface and the hands are in an overhand grip position while being approximately shoulder width apart on the hoop.

PERFORMANCE
Lift/swing the hoop upward, overhead, and downward in front of the body. As the hoop passes below the level of the knees, jump directly upward to allow the hoop to travel under the feet. After the hoop travels under the feet, begin to lift/swing the hoop upward behind the body. Land in a bent leg, relaxed position on the balls of the feet inside the hoop. The hands are positioned directly in front of the hips and the hoop continues its upward then overhead movement. Repeat the procedure to continue Hoop Jumping Forward.

DESCRIPTION
Hold the hoop while being inside the hoop with an overhand grip.
Lift/swing the hoop upward, overhead, and downward in front of the body.
Jump the hoop as it passes under the feet.
Lift/swing the hoop upward then overhead to repeat the procedure.

ADDITIONAL TEACHING SUGGESTIONS

1) Demonstrate and discuss the skill. Break the skill down into its component parts.

2) Introduce the skill in a whole/part and part/whole teaching technique progression.

3) Stress the importance of having one's personal space and staying within the personal space.

4) Encourage the students to use the overhand grip.

5) Make certain the students keep their hands approximately shoulder width apart on the hoop.

6) Emphasize the need to keep the chin level and the shoulders back throughout the entire performance of the skill. Allowing the chin to drop and the shoulders to move forward results in loss of balance and the opportunity for the student to fall.

7) Stress the proper landing technique: bend knees, keep chin level, and land on balls of feet.

8) Discuss the movement of the hands and wrists to allow the hoop to travel in the circular pathway.

9) Challenge the students to continue to perform Hoop Jumping Forward without stopping.

10) Have the students perform different styles of jumping/passing over the hoop, single jump, rebound/double jump, hop, gallop, skip, etc.

11) Use students who are successful with the skill to assist those students who need additional assistance. Stress cooperation, human worth and dignity, and compassion.

12) Give the students opportunities to demonstrate the skill. Have classmates clap for the demonstrators.

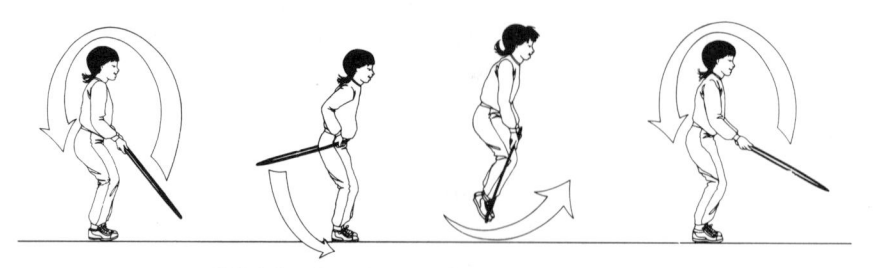

HOOP JUMPING BACKWARD

<u>STARTING POSITION</u>
Begin in a bent leg, relaxed standing position with the feet together. The arms are extended downward with the hands grasping the hoop at mid thigh level. The hoop is positioned diagonally downward and the hands are in an underhand grip position while being approximately shoulder width apart on the hoop.

PERFORMANCE

List/swing the hoop upward, overhead, and downward to place the body inside the hoop. As the hoop passes below the level of the knees, jump directly upward to allow the hoop to travel under the feet. After the hoop travels under the feet, begin to lift/swing the hoop upward in front of the body. Land in a bent leg, relaxed position on the balls of the feet. The hands are positioned directly in front of the hips and the hoop continues its upward then overhead movement. Repeat the procedure to continue Hoop Jumping Backward.

DESCRIPTION

Hold the hoop in front of the body with an underhand grip.
Lift/swing the hoop upward and overhead.
Swing the hoop downward with the body inside the hoop.
Jump the hoop as it passes under the feet.
Lift/swing the hoop upward then overhead to repeat the procedure.

ADDITIONAL TEACHING SUGGESTIONS

1) Demonstrate and discuss the skill. Break the skill down into its component parts.

2) Introduce the skill in a whole/part and part/whole teaching technique progression.

3) Stress the importance of having one's personal space and staying within the personal space.

4) Encourage the students to use the underhand grip.

5) Make certain the students keep their hands approximately shoulder width apart on the hoop.

6) Emphasize the need to keep the chin level and the shoulders back throughout the entire performance of the skill. Allowing the chin to drop and the shoulders to move forward results in a loss of balance and the opportunity for the student to fall. .

7) Stress the proper landing technique: bend knees, keep chin level, and land on balls of feet.

8) Discuss the movement of the hands and wrists to allow the hoop to travel in the circular pathway.

9) Challenge the students to continue to perform Hoop Jumping Backward without stopping.

10) Have the students perform different styles of jumping/passing over the hoop: single jump, rebound/double jump, hop, gallop, skip, etc.

11) Use students who are successful with the skill to assist those students who need additional assistance. Stress cooperation, human worth and dignity, and compassion.

12) Give the students opportunities to demonstrate the skill. Have classmates clap for the demonstrators.

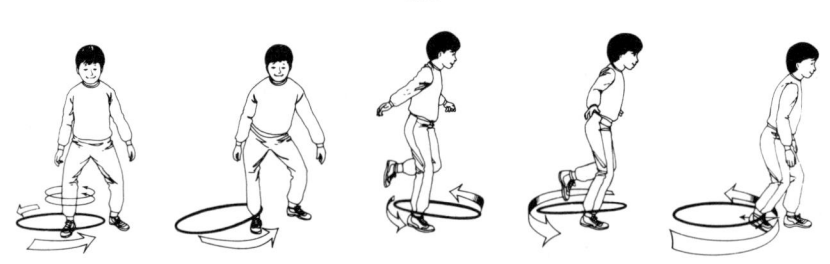

HOOP TWIRL ON ANKLE

STARTING POSITION
Stand in a relaxed position with the feet slightly greater than shoulder width apart. The dominate foot is inside the hoop with the front of the hoop sitting on top of the dominate foot.

PERFORMANCE
Circle the dominate foot in a counterclockwise direction by sliding the foot across the floor to begin the twirl of the hoop around the ankle. As the hoop passes the front of the dominate foot, lift the opposite foot to allow the hoop to pass under the foot. Immediately after the hoop passes under the opposite foot, lower the foot to the floor. Continue to have the hoop twirl around the dominate ankle by moving the dominate foot forward and backward. In the process, lift the opposite foot each time the hoop twirls past the front of the dominate foot to allow the hoop to continue its twirl by passing under the opposite foot.

DESCRIPTION
Stand with the dominate foot inside the hoop.
Place the hoop on top of the dominate foot.
Circle the dominate foot in a counterclockwise direction.
Lift the opposite foot to allow the twirling hoop to pass beneath it.
Lower the opposite foot to floor.
Move the dominate foot forward and backward.
Continue to step over the twirling hoop with the opposite foot.

ADDITIONAL TEACHING SUGGESTIONS

1) Demonstrate and discuss the skill. Break the skill down into its component parts.

2) Introduce the skill in a whole/part and part/whole teaching technique progression.

3) Stress the importance of having one's personal space and staying within the personal space.

4) Emphasize the need to begin the skill with the hoop placed on top of the dominate foot.

5) Make certain the students begin the hoop twirl by circling the dominate foot in a counterclockwise direction.

6) Discuss the timing of the hoop twirl around the dominate ankle to be able to step over the twirling hoop with the opposite foot.

7) Continue to emphasize the need to move the dominate foot forward and backward following the initial circling of the dominate foot to allow the hoop to continuously twirl around the dominate ankle.

8) Use students who are successful with the skill to assist those students who need additional assistance. Stress cooperation, human worth and dignity, and compassion.

9) Give the students opportunities to demonstrate the skill. Have classmates clap for the demonstrators.

Chapter Three
ADDITIONAL MANIPULATIVE INDIVIDUAL HOOP SKILLS

1) Have the students walk into open spaces throughout the activity area while rolling their hoops beside them. Instruct the students to travel forward, backward, sideward, and in circles. During the movements, challenge each student to maintain continual contact with the rolling hoop.

2) Tell the students to push their hoops in a forward direction into open spaces. Challenge each student to move in a safe and controlled manner to catch the hoop before it stops rolling. After the student catches the hoop, have the student roll the hoop into another open space and move to catch it.

3) While standing in an open space, have each student hold the hoop in front of the body in a vertical position so the hoop touches the floor. On a signal, have each student release the hoop and try to pass through the hoop before the hoop falls to the floor. Continue to repeat the process. Ask the students to perform the skill on their own if they can handle the responsibility. As an extension, give students the opportunity to roll their hoops toward open spaces and attempt to carefully crawl through their own rolling hoop. Make certain the hoops roll into open spaces and closely monitor the students as they pass through the hoops. Do not permit the students to dive through the hoops. This activity may not be appropriate for every student or every group of students.

4) Have the students place themselves inside their hoops with the hoop touching the back of the knees. Toss the hoop in a circular direction and immediately begin to bend the knees forward and backward in an attempt to have the hoop twirl around the knees. During the knee movements, keep the feet in place and the body in a balanced upright position.

5) As an extension of Hoop Twirl On The Neck and Hoop Twirl On The Waist, start with the Hoop Twirl On The Neck. As the hoop twirls around the neck, extend one arm upward through the hoop then immediately extend the other arm upward through the hoop to allow the hoop to twirl downward around the upper arms, shoulders, and chest. When the hoop twirls past the chest, start forward/backward or sideward movements with the hips to have the hoop stop its downward movement and begin to Hoop Twirl On The Waist.

6) As an extension of the Hoop Twirl On The Waist and the Hoop Twirl On The Knees, start with the Hoop Twirl On The Waist. While the hoop twirls around the waist, begin to slow down the hip movements to allow the hoop to twirl downward across the buttocks and thighs. When the hoop twirls past the thighs, start forward and backward movements with the knees to have the hoop stop its downward movement and begin to Hoop Twirl On The Knees.

7) Perform the Hoop Twirl On The Wrist with the arm extended upward. Perform the skill on each wrist. Exchange the hoop from wrist to wrist.

8) Perform the Hoop Twirl On The Wrist. As the hoop twirls in an upward direction around the wrist, lift the arm and toss the hoop into the air while quickly pulling the wrist/hand out of the hoop. Watch the path of the hoop and the twirling movement. Extend the hand/wrist into the twirling hoop when the hoop falls in front of the body. Begin the Hoop Twirl On The Wrist by circling the wrist/hand in the direction of the twirl then begin the upward/downward movement of the wrist/hand. Perform the skill on each wrist then perform the skill by tossing the hoop from wrist to wrist. As an extension, toss the hoop in the air, turn around, catch the hoop on the wrist, and begin the Hoop Twirl On The Wrist.

9) Have the students place their hoops in open spaces on the ground surface throughout the activity area. While positioning the feet shoulder width apart, instruct each student to place one foot inside the hoop. Without moving the feet, tell each student to lift the hoop off the floor to take the hoop from one side of the body to the other side of the body while having the body pass through the hoop. Repeat the procedure in the other direction.

10) After the students scatter into open spaces throughout the activity area, instruct each student to circle the hoop around the waist by performing hand-offs in front of and in back of the body. Repeat the activity by circling the hoop in the other direction. As an extension, challenge each student to circle the hoop around different body parts: neck, chest, knees, and ankles. Also, vary the speed and continually change the body part to circle.

11) Perform the Hoop Twirl On The Wrist. As the hoop twirls on the wrist, make a 180° turn and extend the other arm/wrist behind the body to place the wrist/hand inside the twirling hoop. Take the initial wrist/hand out of the twirling hoop and begin to twirl the hoop on the other wrist/hand and complete the full turn. If successful, challenge the students to perform the hoop exchange by turning in the other direction.

Chapter Four
INDIVIDUAL ACTIVITIES WITH THE HOOP IN AN OPEN SPACE ON THE FLOOR

1) Perform locomotor movements around the outside of the hoop; walk, march, jog, run, jump, hop, gallop, skip, slide, etc. Travel in both directions: clockwise and counterclockwise. Make certain the movements are away from the hoop. Use a rhythmical accompaniment; wood block, dance drum, triangle, hand clap, etc.

2) Perform locomotor movements near the center of the hoop; march, jog, run, jump, hop and skip. Caution the students about staying near the center. Do not permit the students to step on the hoop. Use a rhythmical accompaniment; wood block, dance drum, triangle, hand clap, etc.

3) Have the students practice and reinforce directional concepts through a variety of teaching styles and approaches such as:

a) Stand inside your hoop.

b) Can you carefully step over your hoop to place yourself outside the hoop?

c) Who can find a safe way to move around the hoop while traveling at a low level? Medium level? High level?

d) Balance on one foot beside your hoop.

e) On the count of three, let's stand so that our hoops are behind us....ready; 1, 2, 3.

f) Place your body under your hoop.

g) How many different ways can you find to safely pass through your hoop?

h) Let's stand beside our hoops. Now, safely step sideward over your hoop to place yourself inside your hoop.

i) While always returning safely to the inside of your hoop, let's step out of our hoops while traveling in different directions; forward, backward, sideward, to the right, to the left, etc.

j) I bet you can't think of a safe way to place your body above your hoop at a low level? Medium level? High level?

k) As I show you a word card, perform the directional movement shown without touching your hoop while traveling outside your hoop. On my command, let's always safely return to the inside of our hoops so another directional movement card can be shown.

l) Can you find at least five safe ways to move from the inside to the outside of your hoop. If you like someone else's idea, try it!

m) Let's play the game called "Simon Says" to practice our directional movements. Please remember, only move if Simon says to move. Count the number of times you move when Simon tells you to move. We'll find out how well you did at the end of our game.

n) How many boys and girls know the rhyme called "Jack Be Nimble"? Let's play a game while saying the verse. We'll say the first part of the rhyme together, then I will give you the directional movement to perform. Ready, "Jack be nimble, Jack be quick, Jack...step into your hoop." Again, "Jack be nimble, Jack be quick, Jack...step to the right to leave your hoop." After a number of teacher directed commands, give the students opportunities to finish the verse.

4) Perform Fun Stunts around the outside of the hoop; crab walk (forward, backward and sideward), seal walk, bear walk, lame puppy dog walk, double lame puppy dog walk, inchworm, elephant walk, bunny rabbit jump, frog jump, and army crawl.

5) Have the students hold balance or statue positions on a specific number of body parts inside the hoop, outside the hoop, or inside/outside the hoop. For example, challenge the students to...."Find a safe balance position on three body parts inside the hoop or create a safe statue position on two body parts outside the hoop." As an extension, challenge the students to create the balance or statue position at a specific level; low, medium or high.

6) Have the students hold balance or statue positions on specific body parts inside the hoop, outside the hoop, or inside/outside the hoop. For example, challenge the students to...."Find a safe balance position on one hand inside the hoop and on both feet outside the hoop or create a safe statue position on one hand and one foot inside the hoop and on one knee outside the hoop." As an extension, challenge the students to create the balance or statue position at a specific level; low, medium, or high.

7) Instruct the students to kick then chase their hoops. Emphasize safe and controlled kicks so the hoops stay on the ground surface. As a follow-up, have the students begin by kicking their own hoop then proceed to give up their own hoop and start kicking other hoops. Again, stress safe and controlled kicks.

8) Give the students a basketball or one of comparable size. Ask the students to dribble the ball around their hoop in a counterclockwise direction using the right hand. Repeat the activity by traveling in a clockwise direction while dribbling the ball with the left hand. Continue the activity by having the students dribble the ball inside their hoop; dominate hand, opposite hand, and alternate hands at different levels of high, medium and low. As an extension, instruct the students to dribble the ball around their hoop in a specific direction and on a signal, have the students leave their hoop to dribble the ball to another hoop, then continue to dribble the ball around the new hoop in the same direction.

9) Give each student a hoop and a bean bag. Ask each student to place the hoop in an open space against the wall. In the beginning, have each student start with their toes touching the hoop and take one step backward. Toss the bean bag into the hoop using the proper underhand throw. After all students have tossed their bean bags, have the students retrieve their bean bags and repeat the process by taking two steps backward. Continue the activity by increasing the number of backward steps by one each time. Limit the number of steps according to the grade level and/or ability levels of the students and the availability of sufficient space to keep the activity safe and under control. Repeat the activity and have the students toss the bean bags into the hoop using the proper overhand throw. Consider starting with five steps backward. If possible, allow the students practice time to continue the activity by giving them the flexibility to set their own distances and to choose the throw to use. Monitor the students closely to make certain they are establishing realistic distances and are staying on task.

10) Give each student a hoop and a ball. Change the size of the ball each time the activity is repeated. Ask each student to place the hoop in an open space against the wall. In the beginning, have each student start with their toes touching the hoop and take one step backward. While using the underhand throw, gently toss the ball at a low level against the wall so that it will bounce inside the hoop, and catch it off the first bounce. After a specific number of successful throws and catches, have each student or the total group of students slide the hoop a specific distance away from the wall. Continue to repeat this procedure. Consider placing distance markings on the floor in front of the wall for the students to use during the process. As the hoop moves away from the wall, it will be necessary to discuss the differences in the tosses since each toss will have to be higher with more intensity. Be certain to stop the movement of the hoop away from the wall when the distance reaches a point in which the students are not being successful. Keep the activity under control. As a modification, repeat the activity and have the students catch the ball off a specific numbered bounce. Begin with two bounces and repeat the backward movement of the hoop after a specific number of successful tosses and catches. Start the activity again by having the students catch the ball after three bounces.

11) Give each student a hoop and a ball. Change the size of the ball each time the activity is repeated. Ask each student to place the hoop in an open space against the wall. In the beginning, have each student start with their toes touching the hoop and take two steps backward. While using the underhand throw or a modified overhand throw carefully toss the ball into the hoop so it bounces off the floor then off the wall. Catch the ball of the wall. After a specific number of successful throws and catches, have the student or the total group of students slide the hoop a specific distance away from the wall. Continue to repeat this procedure. Consider placing distance markings on the floor in front of the wall for the students to use during the process. As the hoop moves away from the wall, it will be necessary to discuss the difference in the tosses since each toss will have to have more intensity/speed. Be certain to stop the movement of the hoop away from the wall when the distance reaches a point in which the students are not being successful. Keep the activity under control. As a modification, repeat the activity and have the students catch the ball off the first bounce from the ground surface (inside the hoop/wall/ground surface/catch). Repeat the backward movement of the hoop after a specific number of successful tosses and catches. Start the activity again by having the students catch the ball after two bounces.

12) Have the students perform the Hokey Pokey dance using their individual hoop. Instruct the students to place specific body parts and the whole self inside their hoop so as not to touch the hoop. In particular, have the student carefully step into their hoop and out of their hoop to perform the "whole self" segment of the dance. <u>Do not</u> permit the students to step on their hoop.

13) Give each student one of the following; a set of number cards (1 to 10), a variety of colored square pieces of paper, a set of alphabet letter cards, or a variety of paper shapes. Instruct the students to place a specific item (number 10 card, yellow square, letter B, or a triangle) in the center of the hoop then perform a specific locomotor movement around the hoop. During the performance of the locomotor movement, quickly move throughout the scattered hoops to assess the requested task. After the quick assessment, stop the students and have them remove the item from the hoop. Continue the activity by having the students place another item from a specific group of cards in the center and perform a different locomotor movement around the hoop. As an extension, have the students solve a math problem or spell a word. For example, write a math problem on a portable chalkboard or on a large piece of paper and have the students compute the problem then place a number card or number cards in the center of the hoop to record the answer. If the activity involves the set of alphabet letter cards, say a word and have the students pick out the appropriate letters and place the letters in the correct order in the center of the hoop to spell the word. Once again, after the completion of the task, instruct the students to perform a locomotor movement around the hoop and quickly assess the completion of the task.

14) Give each student a ball. Have the students perform a variety of basic ball handling skills including: drop the ball into the hoop and catch the ball at head level, shoulder level, chest level, waist level, knee level, and ankle level while standing outside the hoop; toss the ball into the air directly above the hoop and catch the ball off the first bounce, second bounce, third bounce, etc., while standing outside the hoop; and toss the ball into the air directly above the hoop and clap the hands one time before catching the ball in the air or off the first bounce then continue the activity by adding one clap each time the prior task was successfully completed.

15) Instruct the students to position their bodies in a side leaning rest position with the body being supported on one straightened arm with the hand placed near the center of the hoop. The other arm and hand is positioned against the side of the body. While maintaining the side leaning rest position, instruct the students to walk around the extended arm while turning the hand in place. The traveling is done on the sides of the feet. Relate the activity to the Fun Stunt called "Coffee Grinder." Repeat the activity supporting the body on the other hand and traveling in the other direction. As an extension, have the students begin in a push-up position with the hands placed near the center of the hoop. Repeat the procedure of traveling around the hoop by taking side steps with the feet while continually repositioning the hands as the body travels around the hoop. Repeat the activity by traveling in the other direction.

Chapter Five
PARTNER ACTIVITIES WITH THE HOOP IN AN OPEN SPACE ON THE FLOOR

1) Perform locomotor movements around the outside of the hoop while being one behind the other or one beside the other with the inside hands joined; walk, march, jog, run, jump, hop, gallop, skip, slide, etc. Travel in both directions: clockwise and counterclockwise. Make certain the movements are away from the hoop. Use a rhythmical accompaniment; wood block, dance drum, triangle, hand clap, etc.

2) Have the students combine their bodies together in safe and controlled balance or statue positions on a specific number of body parts inside the hoop, outside the hoop, or inside/outside the hoop. For example, challenge the students to...."Find a safe balance position on five combined body parts inside the hoop or create a safe statue position on three body parts inside the hoop and on two body parts outside the hoop." As an extension, challenge the students to create the balance or statue position at a specific level; low, medium, high, or at a combination of two levels.

3) Have the students combine their bodies together in safe and controlled balance or statue positions on specific body parts inside the hoop, outside the hoop, or inside/outside the hoop. For example, challenge the students to...."Find a safe balance position on three feet and two hands inside the hoop or create a safe statue position on two feet, two hands, and one knee outside the hoop." As an extension, challenge the students to create the balance or statue position at a specific level; low, medium, high, or at a combination of two levels.

4) While staying in open spaces, have the students kick a hoop back and forth. Emphasize safe and controlled kicks so the hoop stays on the ground surface. Tell the students to stop/trap the hoop prior to kicking it back to the partner. If necessary, set a minimum and maximum distance between partners to maintain control and to help keep the partner groups on task. As an extension, challenge the partner groups to attempt to continuously kick the hoop back and forth without stopping/trapping the hoop assuming the partner groups can handle the open ended partner group task.

5) Give each partner group a ball. Vary the size of the ball each time the activity is performed. In the beginning, have each student start with their toes touching the hoop while being directly across from each other. Tell each student to take one step backward. Use the underhand throw and have the students play catch by tossing the ball into the hoop so the partner catches it from a bounce. After a brief practice session, repeat the process by taking two steps backward. Continue the activity by increasing the number of backward steps which will increase the number of bounces before the partner catches the ball. In order to keep the activity safe and under control, limit the number of steps according to the grade level and/or ability levels

of the students and the availability of sufficient activity space. If possible, repeat the activity using the proper overhand throw, however, make certain the group of students is capable of performing the task since the ball travels faster. Also, make certain the students have the ability to accurately throw the ball at a specific target. Have the students begin the overhand throw activity by taking five steps backward from the hoop.

6) Give each partner group one of the following: a set of number cards (1 to 10) or a set of alphabet letter cards. Write a math problem on a portable chalkboard or on a large piece of paper and have the students compute the problem then place a number card or number cards in the center of the hoop to record the answer. If the activity involves the set of alphabet letter cards, say a word and have the students pick out the appropriate letters and place the letters in the correct order in the center of the hoop to spell the word. After the completion of the designated task, allow the students to participate in an individual or partner activity; rope jumping, throwing and catching, manipulative ball skills, etc., until the remaining partner groups complete the task. During the performance of the follow-up activity, quickly move throughout the scattered hoops to assess the requested task. After the quick assessment, stop the students and have them remove the item(s) from the hoops. Continue the activity by giving the students another math problem or a word to spell.

Chapter Six
ACTIVE GAMES AND ACTIVE RELAY RACES

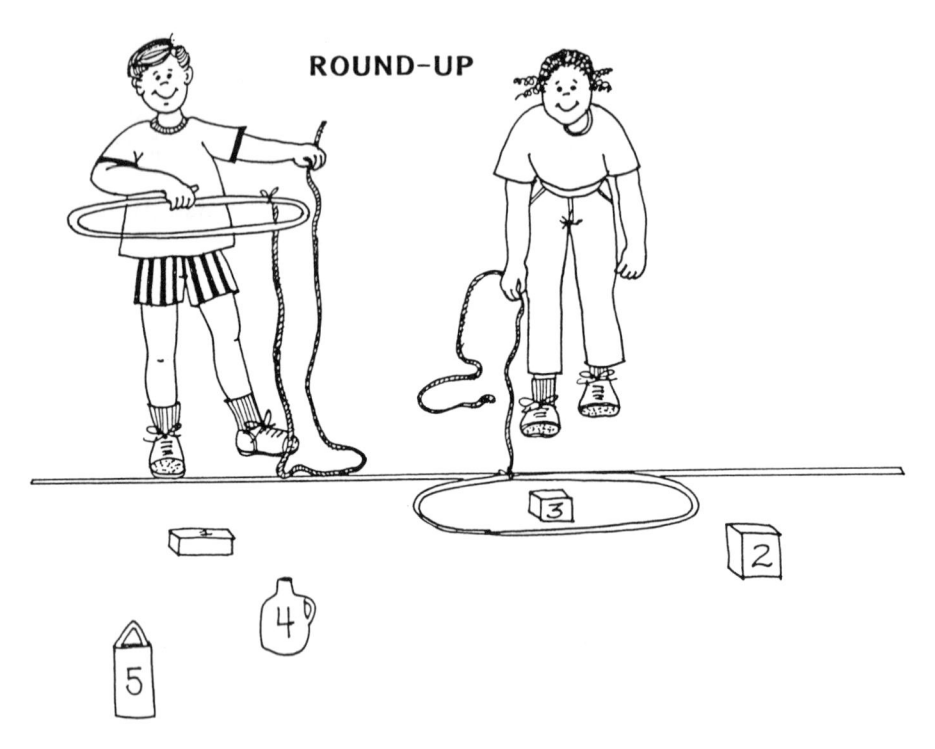

ROUND-UP

Set up a large number of various size boxes, empty milk cartons, or plastic jugs throughout the game activity area in front of a designated foul line. Place a point value on the front of each object and increase the point value of the objects according to their distances from the foul line and the size/shape of the objects. Give each student a hoop with a long rope or cord tied to it. On the starting signal, instruct each student to toss the hoop in an attempt to lasso an object and drag the object across the foul line. Have the students continue to toss the hoops, lasso the objects, and pull the objects across the foul line until the end of the playing time. At the conclusion of the game, have each student count and report their individual score.

ADDITIONAL TEACHING SUGGESTIONS

1) In order to keep the students active and on task, use this game as a station with a small number of participants unless there is enough space and equipment to keep an entire class involved.

2) Make the game cooperative by giving the group of students a designated amount of time to accumulate a specific number of points. If the group is successful, challenge the students to complete the task in a shorter amount of time or increase the number of points.

3) Promote honesty and compliment students' exhibiting honesty throughout the game.

4) Discuss the title of the game and the relationship between the actions within the game to the occurrences within a rodeo.

5) Use students to demonstrate proper throwing and lassoing techniques. Have classmates clap for the demonstrators.

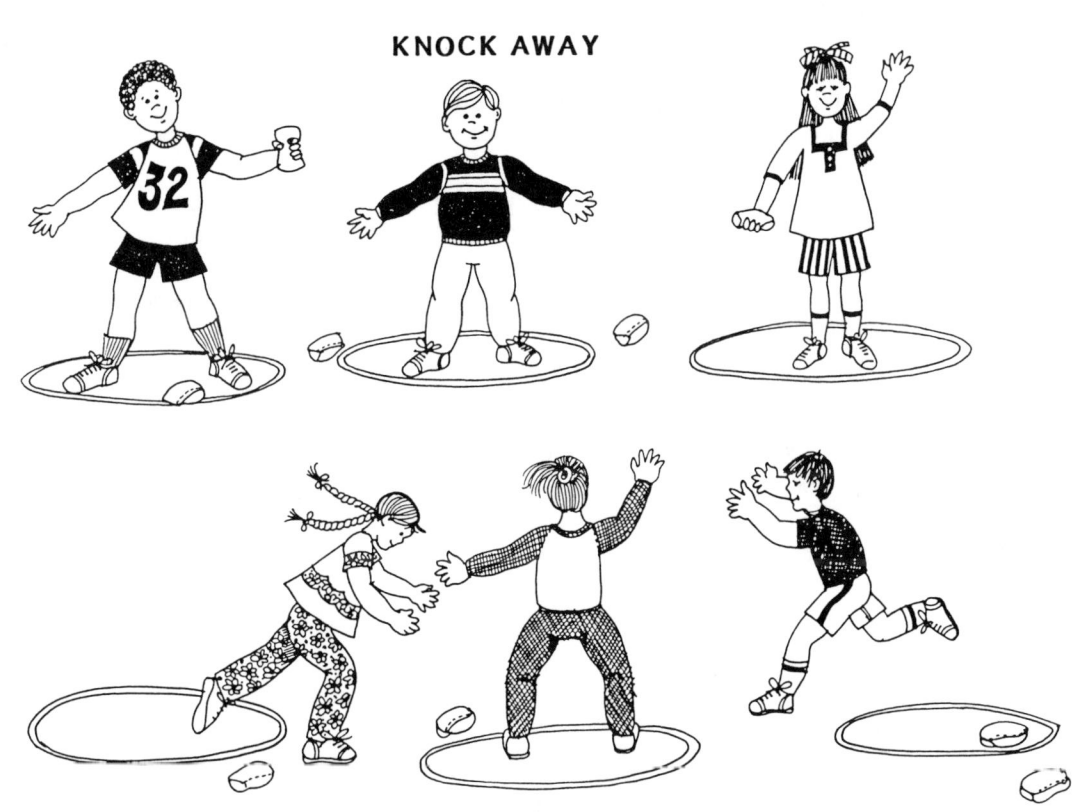

KNOCK AWAY

Organize the students into groups of six. Subdivide each group into two teams of three students. Give each student a hoop and a minimum of three bean bags. Set up separate playing areas for each group of six students. Have the three students from opposing teams place their hoops directly across from each other at a distance of approximately five yards. At the beginning of the game, each student stands in his/her hoop while holding one bean bag. The remaining bean bags are placed on the floor outside the hoop. On the starting signal, the players on each team attempt to toss their bean bags into the opposing teams' hoops using the underhand throw. Players may bat the bean bags to protect their hoop areas or they may catch the bean bags. A point is scored each time a bean bag is thrown in one of the opposing teams' hoops. Players may leave their hoops to retrieve bean bags; however, in so doing, the hoops become unguarded. At the conclusion of the game, have each student share the number of bean bags which were tossed into his or her hoop. Determine the team score by adding the three player's scores.

ADDITIONAL TEACHING SUGGESTIONS

1) Make certain the playing areas for the various groups of six are separate so there is no overlapping between games.

2) Use students to demonstrate proper underhand throw technique. Have classmates clap for the demonstrators.

3) Discuss the need to throw the bean bag at a low level. Stress safety!

4) Establish teams that are coed and equal in ability levels.

5) Provide time for team members to discuss game strategies and team play.

6) Even though the game is competitive and points are scored by opposing teams, consider lessening the importance of the accumulated points. Instead, highlight sportsmanship, honesty in keeping one's score and the final team score, team play, and the individual and team effort presented throughout the game regardless of the outcome of the game.

7) Rotate team players between opposing teams at the conclusion of each game to vary the learning experiences and lessen the competitive feeling.

8) Provide time at the end of the games to allow players the opportunity to share thoughts about the game.

9) As an extension to the school's writing program, provide three to five minutes at the end of a class period for students to put their thoughts on paper. Collect the writings at the end of the lesson. Do not grade the papers or correct grammar. Take the time to read the papers. Return the writings to the students within the next lesson and allow students time to voluntarily read their writings to classmates in informal partner group or small group settings.

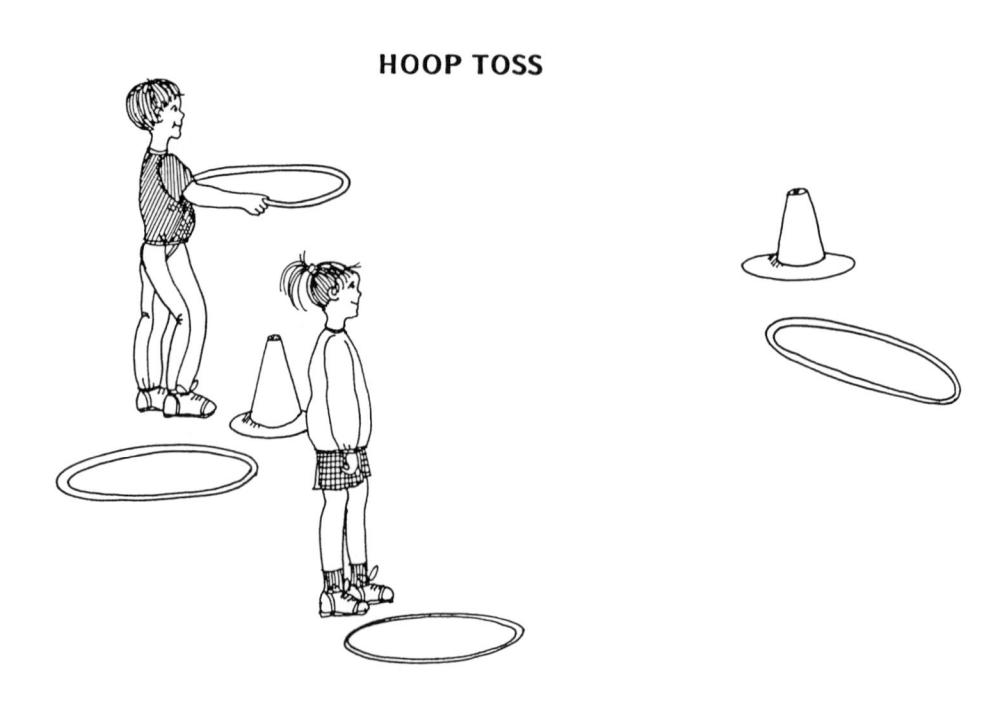

HOOP TOSS

Organize the students into partner groups. Give each partner group two large cones and give each student two medium size hoops. The two sets of hoops have to be different colors. Instruct the students to place the two large cones across from each other at a distance of ten to fifteen feet apart. Both students start on opposite sides of the same cone and alternate tosses toward the other cone in an attempt to score points. After all tosses are made, the students move to the cone to tabulate their scores. Scoring is as follows: three points for a ringer (the hoop completely surrounds the cone), two points for a leaner (the hoop touches or leans against the cone), and one point if the hoop is close to the cone (the distance can't be greater than the diameter of the hoop). After the scores are tabulated, the students repeat the throwing procedure by tossing the hoops toward the other cone. The first student to reach twenty-one points wins the game.

ADDITIONAL TEACHING SUGGESTIONS

1) Discuss the similarities of the game to the game of horseshoes.

2) Establish partner groups that are equal in ability levels.

3) Provide paper and pencils for the partner groups to use to keep an ongoing tabulation of individual scores.

4) Increase or decrease the distance between the two cones to meet the ability levels of the various groups of students. Allow each group to establish their own "realistic" distance, if possible.

5) Use students to demonstrate proper throwing technique. Have classmates clap for the demonstrators.

6) Have the students within each partner group shake hands or display another acceptable form of sportsmanship at the conclusion of each game.

7) Allow students to change partners at the conclusion of games in order to play other students.

8) Discuss the positive aspects of competition.

9) Set up a ladder tournament for students who are interested. Instead of playing the game to twenty-one points, stop the game after three to five minute intervals. The student who is ahead at the end of the time limit is the winner. If the score is tied, allow one more opportunity to throw the hoops to break the tie.

FRISBEE HULABEE

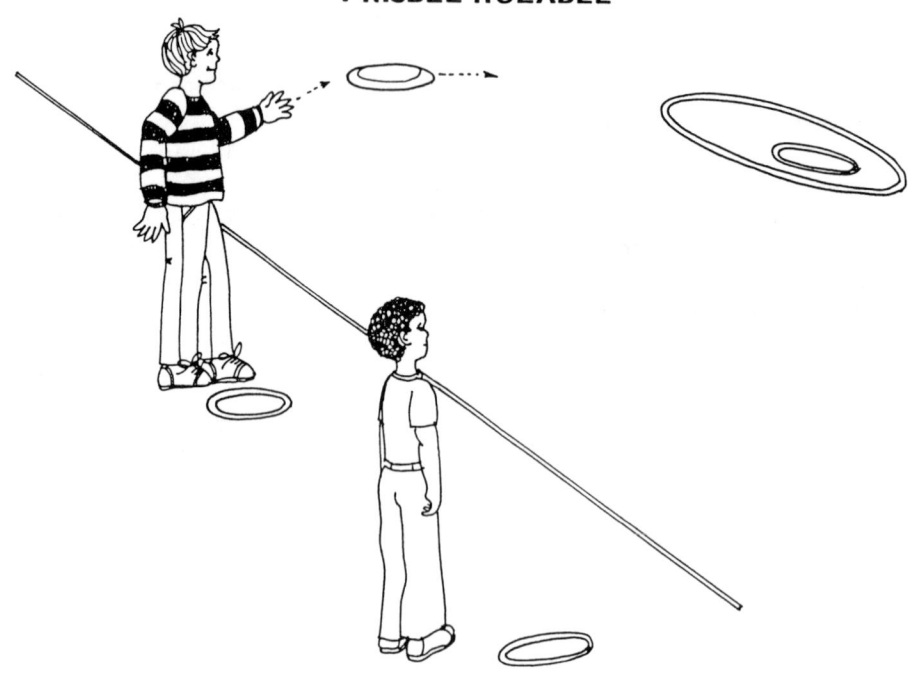

Organize the students into partner groups. Give each partner group one large hoop and four frisbees. The four frisbees need to be in sets of two with contrasting colors because each student gets two frisbees. Instruct each partner group to place the hoop flat on the playing surface fifteen feet in front of the foul line. Each student stands behind the foul line and alternates tosses toward the hoop in an attempt to score points. After all four tosses are made, the students move to the hoop to tabulate their scores. Scoring is as follows: three points for a frisbee that is completely inside the hoop, two points for a frisbee that is touching or on top of part of the hoop, and one point if the frisbee is close to the hoop. The distance can't be greater than the diameter of the frisbee. After the scores are tabulated, the students return to the foul line and repeat the throwing procedure. The first student to reach twenty-one points wins the game.

ADDITIONAL TEACHING SUGGESTIONS

1) Discuss the similarities of the game to the game of horseshoes.

2) Establish partner groups that are equal in ability levels.

3) Provide paper and pencils for the partner groups to use to keep an ongoing tabulation of individual scores.

4) Increase or decrease the distance of the hoop from the foul line to meet the ability levels of the various groups of students. Allow each group to establish their own "realistic" distance, if possible.

5) Play the game as a follow-up activity to a lesson or lessons in which proper frisbee throwing and catching instruction was given.

6) Use students to demonstrate proper throwing technique. Have classmates clap for the demonstrators.

7) Have the students within each partner group shake hands or display another acceptable form of sportsmanship at the conclusion of each game.

8) Allow students to change partners at the conclusion of games to play other students.

9) Discuss the positive aspects of competition.

10) Set up a ladder tournament for students who are interested. Instead of playing the game to twenty-one points, stop the games after three to five minute intervals. The student who is ahead at the end of the time limit is the winner. If the score is tied, allow one more opportunity to throw the frisbees to break the tie.

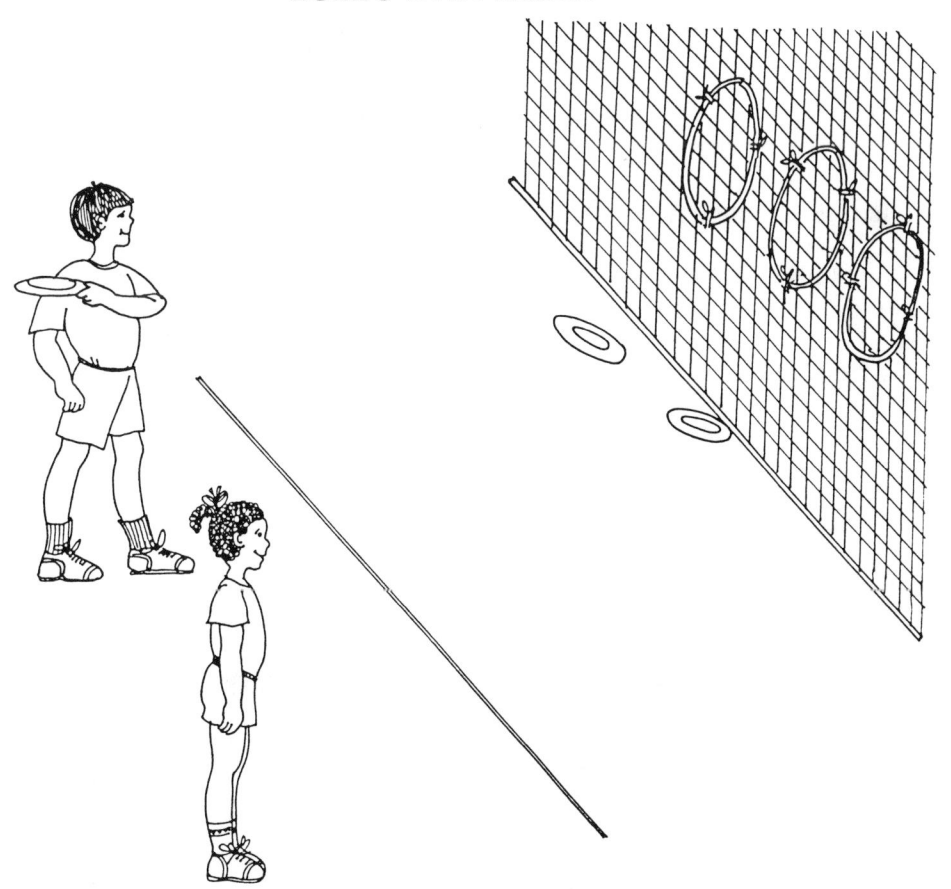

BULL'S-EYE FRISBEE

Organize the students into partner groups. Give each partner group three frisbees. Assign each partner group to a game area consisting of three suspended hoops positioned beside each other and a foul line placed fifteen to twenty feet from the suspended hoops. The two students stand behind the foul line. One student begins the game by throwing the three frisbees, one at a time, in an attempt to have them pass into the hoops. After the three throws are made, the students move to the hoops to tabulate the score. Scoring is as follows: two points for a frisbee that passes into the center hoop and one point for a frisbee that passes into a side hoop. After the score is tabulated, the students return to the foul line and the second student repeats the process of throwing the frisbees toward the hoops. The first student to reach twenty-one points wins the game.

ADDITIONAL TEACHING SUGGESTIONS

1) Establish partner groups that are equal in ability levels.

2) Provide paper and pencils for the partner groups to use to keep an on-going tabulation of individual scores.

3) Increase or decrease the distance of the foul line from the suspended hoops to meet the ability levels of the various groups of students. Allow each group to establish their own "realistic" distance, if possible.

4) Play the game as a follow-up activity to a lesson or lessons in which proper frisbee throwing and catching instruction was given.

5) Use students to demonstrate proper throwing technique. Have classmates clap for the demonstrators.

6) Give partner groups the opportunity to establish their own point value system for the three suspended hoops.

7) Have the students within each partner group shake hands or display another acceptable form of sportsmanship at the conclusion of each game.

8) Allow students to change partners at the conclusion of games to play other students.

9) Discuss the positive aspects of competition.

10) Set up a ladder tournament for students who are interested. Instead of playing the game to twenty-one points, stop the game after three to five minute intervals. The student who is ahead at the end of the time limit is the winner. If the score is tied, allow one more opportunity to throw the frisbees to break the tie.

SHUFFLE BALL

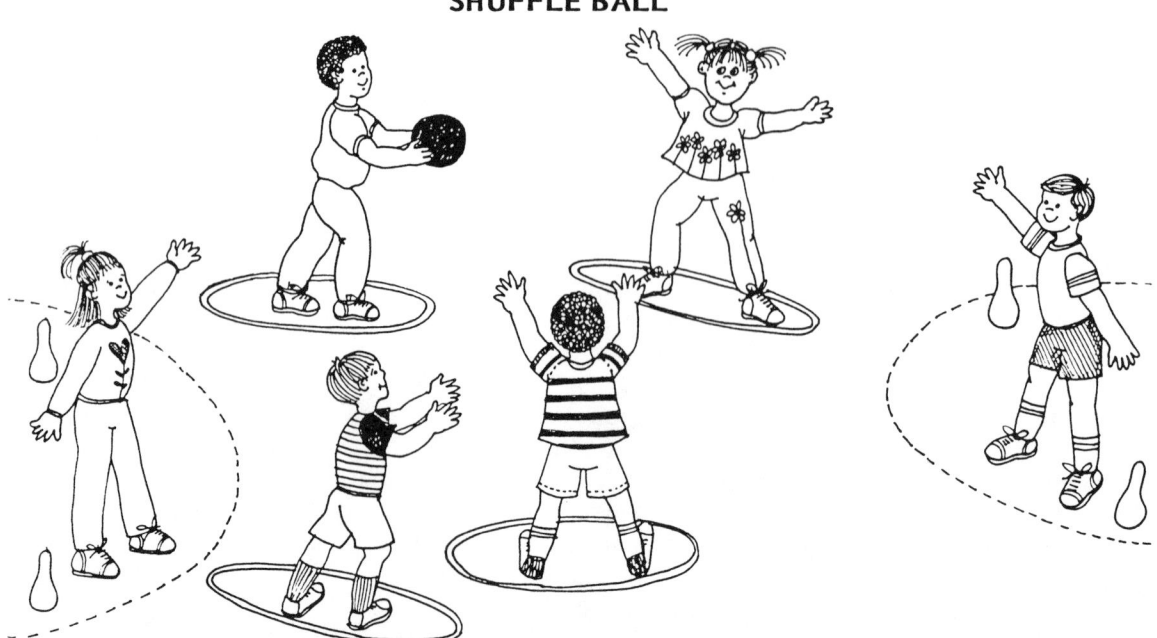

Organize the students into groups of six or eight. Subdivide each group into two teams of equal numbers. Set up playing areas on a hard surface area such as the gymnasium floor, outdoor multipurpose court, tennis courts, etc. Each playing area must contain opposing goalie/crease zones approximately 30 to 40 yards apart. The zone areas are designated by marked half circles with a fifteen foot diameter. Within the goalie-/crease zone is a goalie. It is the goalie's responsibility to protect two plastic bowling pins or similar objects which are set up ten feet apart centered at the back of the half circle. The other team players position themselves near the center of the playing area at the start of the game. These players are not permitted within the goalie-/crease zones. Each player is standing in the middle of a hoop which is lying flat on the playing surface. These players must move/shuffle around the playing area without stepping out of the hoops to move themselves and the hoops. One center player is given a ball. On the signal for the game to begin, the player with the ball can move with the ball for a maximum of three seconds, pass the ball to a fellow teammate, or throw the ball in an attempt to knock down one of the opposing team's pins or objects. During the movement with the ball, the player may dribble the ball or carry the ball. Knocking down a pin/object scores one point and the pin remains down. When the second pin/object is knocked down, a second point is scored and both pins/objects are set up. The members of the winning team rotate positions. The opposing team members repeat the same rotation procedure after their two pins-/objects are knocked down or they, too, can rotate at the conclusion of the game.

PENALTIES

1) If the goalie steps out of the goalie/crease zone, the closest player on the opposing team gets one free throw from the top of the center half circle to knock down a pin/object.

2) If a player steps out of a hoop while controlling the ball, the ball is given to the nearest player on the opposing team.

3) If a player has possession of the ball for more than three seconds, the ball is given to the closest player on the opposing team.

ADDITIONAL TEACHING SUGGESTIONS

1) Establish teams that are coed and equal in ability levels.

2) Use students to referee the games. Rotate students into referee positions, if interested.

3) Discuss the role of the referee and stress the need to show the appropriate respect toward the referee.

4) Provide time for team members to discuss game strategies and team play.

5) Even though the game is competitive and points are scored by opposing teams, consider lessening the importance of the accumulated points. Instead, highlight team play, sportsmanship and fair play, honesty in keeping score, and the individual and team effort displayed throughout the game regardless of the outcome of the game.

6) Have opposing team players line up facing each other at the conclusion of each game, then pass by each other to shake hands or display another form of appropriate sportsmanship behavior.

TARGET TOSS

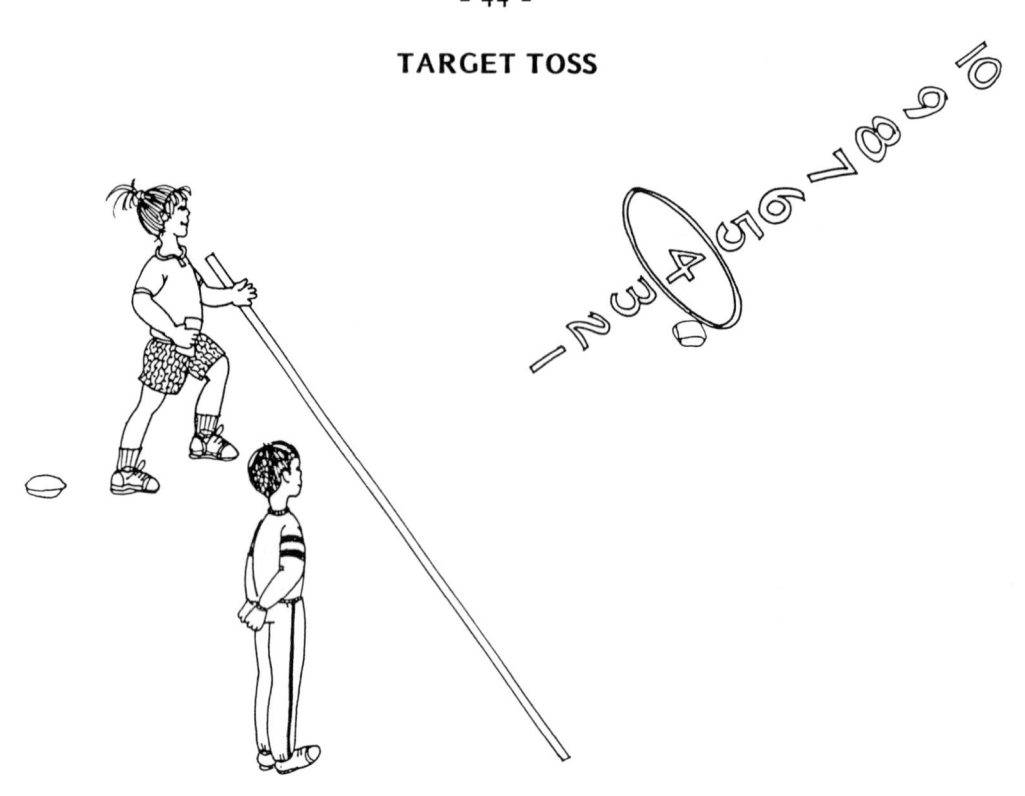

Set up a game activity area which includes a foul line with marked point values on the playing surface extended in a straight line in front of the foul line. The distance between each marked point value is five feet. Start with one point and increase the point value by one point for each additional five foot marker. Divide the students into partner groups and give each partner group one hoop and three bean bags. Have each partner group place their hoop on the first point value marker: one point. Allow each student within a particular group to toss the bean bags, one at a time, from behind the foul line in an attempt to throw the bean bags into the hoop. Points are awarded according to the number of bags landing in the hoop for each point value. For example, if the first student throws two out of three bean bags into the hoop placed on the one point value marker, the student receives two points. After the second student takes his or her turn, the hoop is moved to the second point value marker: two points. If the first student throws one out of three bean bags into the hoop, the student receives two points and the student has accumulated a total of four points. The game continues by placing the hoop on the next point value marker after both students have taken a turn. Points are awarded according to the number of bean bags tossed into the hoop and these points are added to the previous accumulated point value.

After the students in each partner group complete the task of taking turns through the farthest hoop, have them repeat the process in reverse. Move the hoop backward one point value marker toward the foul line. Repeat the process of taking turns to continue scoring points for each point value marker. Continue to accumulate points until both students take turns with the hoop placed on the one point value marker. At the conclusion of the game, instruct each student to share his/her accumulated score with you, and allow the partner group to begin a new game or give permission to each partner group to separate to play the new game with a new partner.

ADDITIONAL TEACHING SUGGESTIONS

1) Review the underhand and overhand throw techniques prior to beginning the game. Discuss the best throw to use according to the distance of the hoop from

the foul line. The underhand throw should be used for short distances and the overhand throw should be used for long distances.

2) Have the thrower stand one step back from the foul line to allow a forward step on the opposite foot during the throwing process so the thrower does not cross the foul line.

3) Instruct the thrower to be responsible for walking to collect the bean bags, then hand them to the partner.

4) Provide paper and pencils for the partner groups to use to keep an ongoing tabulation of individual scores. Have the non-thrower be responsible for keeping score for the thrower.

5) Provide sufficient space between each row of point value markers to permit a safe and unobstructed pathway. Tell the partner groups to travel to the right of their line of point value markers when securing the thrown bean bags.

6) Travel from partner group to partner group to monitor student performance and to check the scoring.

7) Make certain all students take their time while throwing and performing follow-up tasks. <u>Do not</u> allow individual students or partner groups to rush through the tasks to make the completion of the tasks a race within the partner group or between partner groups.

8) Instead of playing the game using the points for competition between the members of each partner group, have each partner group establish a realistic point total to reach and through the combination of individual scores make the activity a cooperative game. If time permits a second game and the partner group met success by reaching the point total, challenge the group to increase their point total. If the point total wasn't reached, have the partner group keep the same point total or decrease the point total to be closer to their combined individual scores/total.

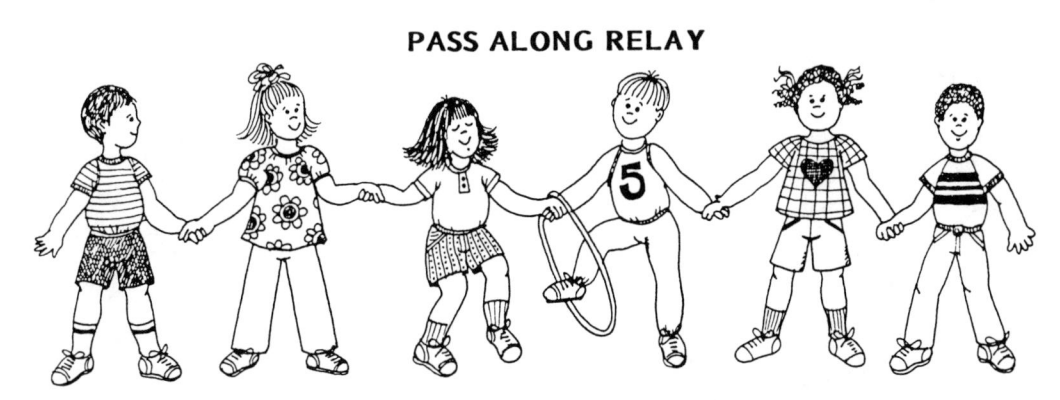

PASS ALONG RELAY

Organize the students into groups of six. Instruct each group of students to stand side by side with hands joined to form a straight line. Give a hoop to the first student in each line. On the starting signal, have the first student pass through the hoop without releasing the grip with the second student. Each student then passes through the hoop in succession. The activity can end after the sixth person goes through the hoop or the activity can continue by repeating the procedure beginning with the sixth student going through the hoop and ending with the first person going through the hoop.

ADDITIONAL TEACHING SUGGESTIONS

1) Discuss cooperation and relate the meaning of the word to the group task to be completed in order to reach success.

2) Set a time limit and challenge each group of students to complete the relay activity before the time expires. Start with a time that allows every group to be successful. Lessen the time for each turn the relay activity is successfully completed. Make certain the time limit is always within a range that is realistically obtainable.

3) Allow time for group interaction before the start of each relay. Permit-/encourage group members to change their order within the line if the group feels the change will help accomplish the task.

4) Modify the relay by increasing or decreasing the number of students on each relay team.

5) Change the formation to a circle and have the group of students go through the hoop to pass it around the circle. Add a second hoop opposite of the first hoop and challenge the students to have the second hoop catch up to the first hoop.

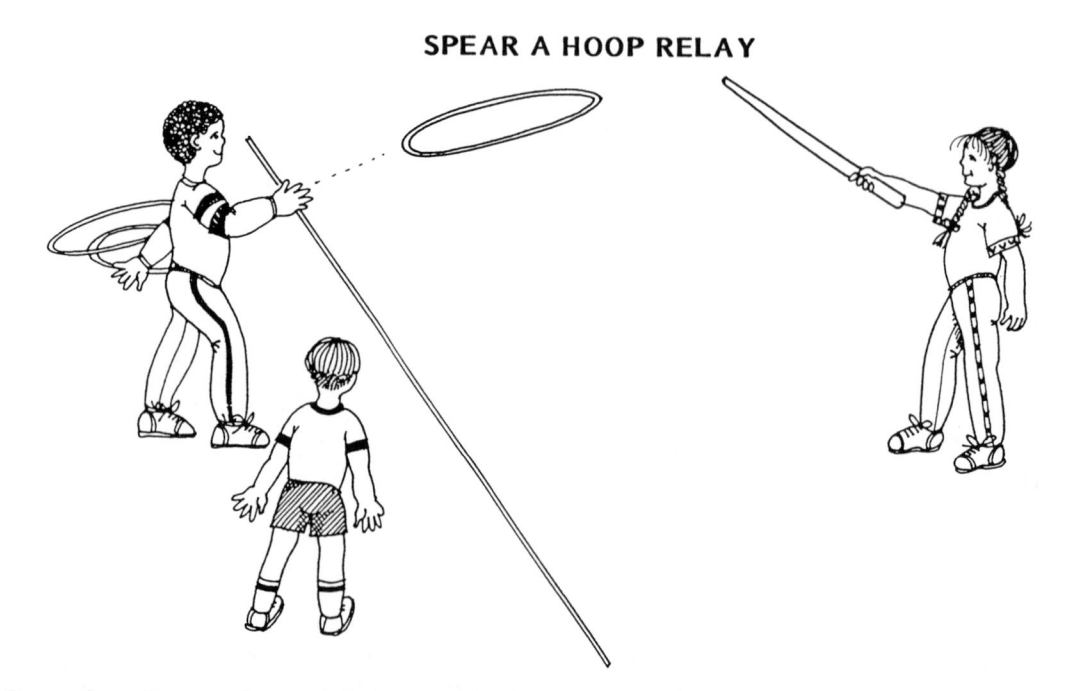

SPEAR A HOOP RELAY

Organize the students into groups of three. Give each group of students a plastic golf tube and four hoops. Have one student from each group stand on a marker ten to fifteen feet in front of the foul line. This student has the plastic tube. The other group members are one behind the other at the foul line. The first student in the line begins the relay by holding one hoop. The remaining three hoops are stacked beside the first student. On the starting signal, the first student in each line carefully tosses the hoop toward the team member with the plastic tube. If the hoop is speared, the team is awarded one point. The first student repeats the procedure with the three remaining hoops. After the first student completes his or her turn, the group members rotate positions. The student who speared the hoops carries the hoops to the foul line and gives them to the next student in the line, then steps behind him or her. The thrower moves forward to be the person to spear the hoops. Points are accumulated among the three team members. The relay is completed when everyone rotates through all three positions.

ADDITIONAL TEACHING SUGGESTIONS

1) Perform the relay as a cooperative activity. Ask each group to establish a number of hoops to be speared. Challenge each group to reach the number. After the relay is completed, have each group repeat the relay by keeping the same number or establishing a higher or lower number based upon the success level of the previous relay.

2) Increase or decrease the distance of the marker from the foul line to meet the ability levels of the various groups of students. Allow each group to establish their own "realistic" distance, if possible.

3) Modify the relay by having the spearer in a kneeling or sitting position.

4) Emphasize the need to carefully toss the hoop so as to not to hit the spearer.

5) Use student demonstrations to show proper throwing and spearing techniques. Have classmates clap for the demonstrators.

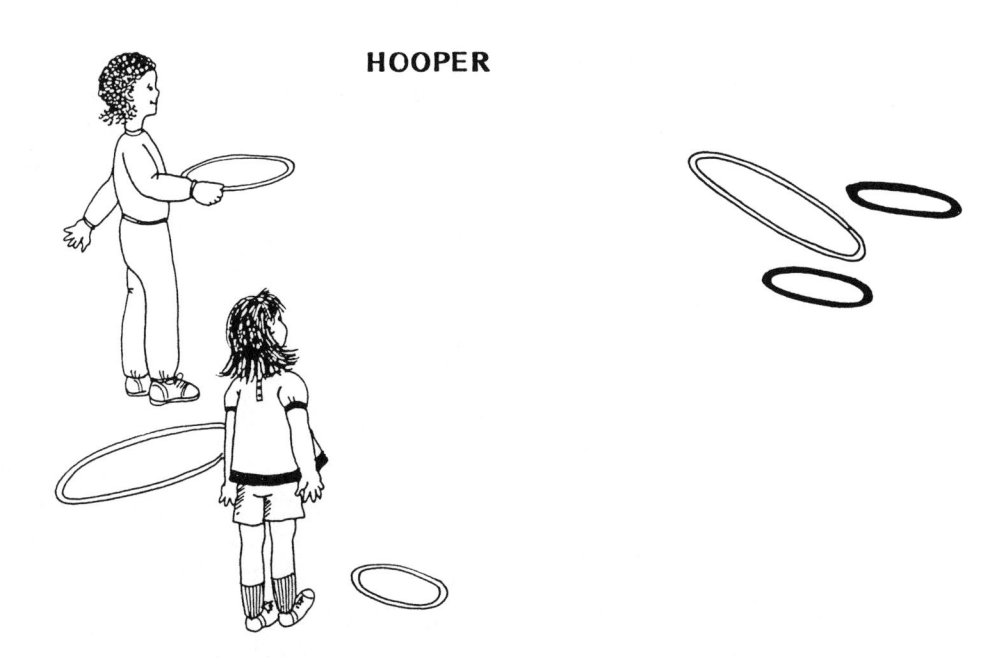

HOOPER

Organize the students into partner groups. Give each partner group two large hoops and give each student two small hoops. The two sets of small hoops have to be different colors. Instruct the students to place the large hoops across from each other at a distance of twenty-five to thirty feet. The students begin the game by standing on opposite sides of one large hoop. Each student tosses their two hoops, one at a time, toward the other large hoop in an attempt to toss the hoops into the large hoop. The students alternate throws. After all tosses are made, the students move to the hoop to tabulate scores. Scoring is as follows: three points for a small hoop inside a large hoop, two points for a small hoop touching or on top of the large hoop, and one point for a small hoop that is close to a large hoop. The distance can't be greater than the diameter of the small hoop. After the scores are tabulated, the students repeat the throwing procedure by tossing the small hoops toward the other large hoop. The first student to reach twenty points wins the game.

ADDITIONAL TEACHING SUGGESTIONS

1) Discuss the similarities of the game to the game of horseshoes.

2) Establish partner groups that are equal in ability levels.

3) Provide paper and pencils for the partner groups to use to keep an ongoing tabulation of individual scores.

4) Increase or decrease the distance between the two large hoops to meet the ability levels of the various groups of students. Allow each group to establish their own "realistic" distance, if possible.

5) Use students to demonstrate proper throwing technique. Have classmates clap for the demonstrators.

6) Have the students within each partner group shake hands or display another acceptable form of sportsmanship at the conclusion of each game.

7) Allow students to change partners at the conclusion of games to play with other students.

8) Discuss the positive aspects of competition.

9) Set up a ladder tournament for students who are interested. Instead of playing the game to twenty points, stop the games after three to five minute intervals. The student who is ahead at the end of the time limit is the winner. If the score is tied, allow one more opportunity to throw the small hoops to break the tie.

HOOP MAZE

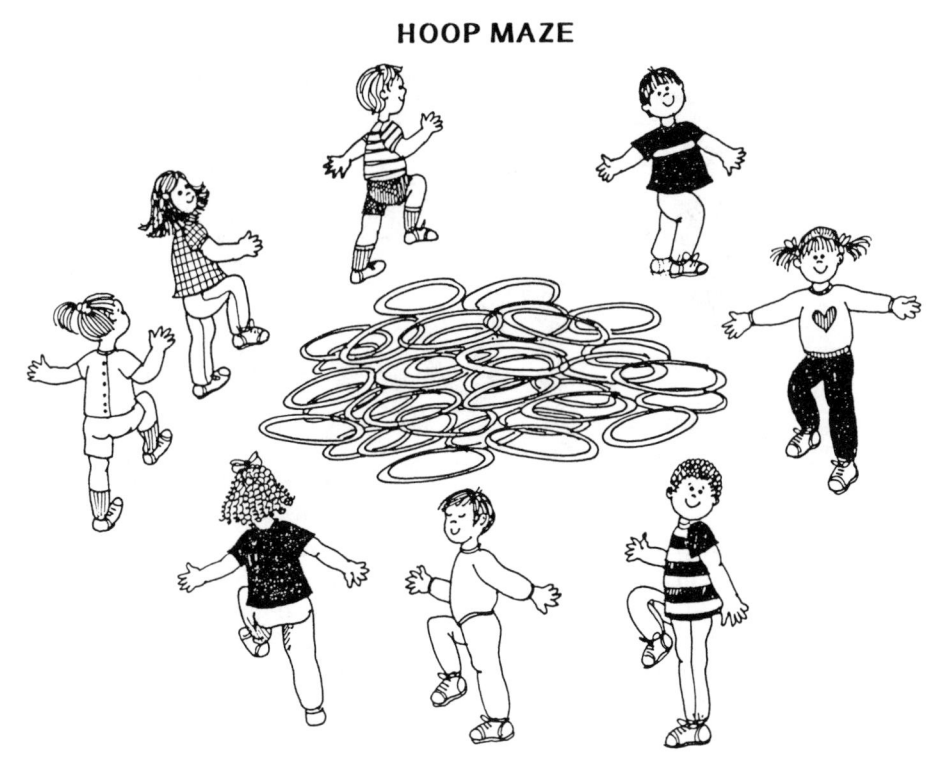

Scatter a large number of hoops in the center of the activity area so the hoops overlap each other. Make certain there are numerous open spaces within the arrangement of the hoops. Ask the students to travel around the pile of hoops performing a specific locomotor movement. On a signal, have the students stop moving and begin to step into the open spaces without touching a hoop or a classmate. After a brief period of time, instruct the students to leave the pile of hoops and continue to move around the pile of hoops while performing a different locomotor movement.

ADDITIONAL TEACHING SUGGESTIONS

1) Explain clockwise and counterclockwise and continually change the direction of movement around the pile of hoops.

2) Ask the students to leave the pile of hoops if a hoop or a classmate is touched. Stress honesty and commend the students for being honest. Allow the students to rejoin the activity during the next movement around the pile of hoops.

3) Modify the game by using partner groups and have the partners move around and throughout the pile of hoops with inside hands joined. Extend this modification by increasing the size of the groups to three, four, or five. Stress cooperation and the need to communicate while traveling through the hoops so as not to touch a hoop or another group of students.

4) Modify the game by giving each student a basketball size ball. Instruct the students to hand dribble the ball while traveling around the pile of hoops. When traveling in a clockwise direction, have the students dribble with the left hand and have the students dribble with the right hand while traveling in a counterclockwise direction. Ask the students to carry the balls while stepping throughout the pile of hoops.

DOWN AND UP RELAY

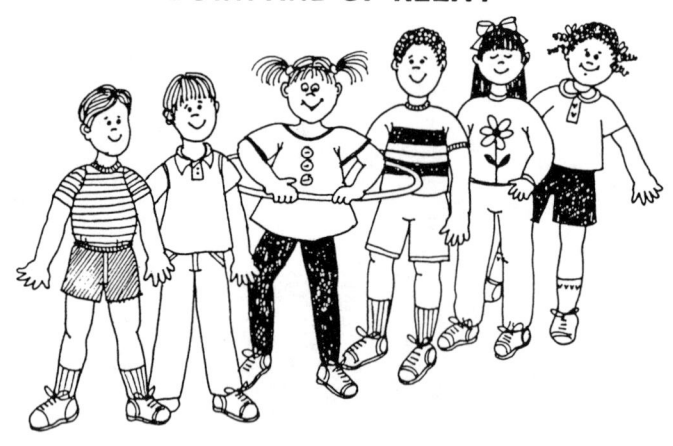

Organize the students into groups of six. Instruct the students in each group to stand one behind the other to form a straight line. Give a hoop to the first student in each line. On the starting signal, the first student takes the hoop down over his or her body (head to feet). Upon completion of the task, the hoop is given to the second student. The second student takes the hoop up over his or her body (feet to head). The relay continues with the remaining four students repeating the sequence of tasks performed by the first two students in the line. The activity can end after the sixth student takes the hoop over his or her body (feet to head) or the activity can continue by repeating the procedure from the sixth student to the first student. If the activity is continued, it ends after the first student passes through the hoop.

ADDITIONAL TEACHING SUGGESTIONS

1) Discuss cooperation and relate the meaning of the word to the group task to be completed in order to reach success.

2) Set a time limit and challenge each group of students to complete the relay activity before the time expires. Start with a time that will allow every group to be successful. Lessen the time for each turn the relay activity is successfully completed. Make certain the time limit is always within a range that is realistically obtainable.

3) Allow time for group interaction before the start of each relay. Permit/encourage group members to change their order within the line if the group feels the change will help accomplish the task.

4) Discuss the need to have sufficient space between each student in the line.

5) Make certain the hand-off from student to student is safe and under control.

6) Modify the relay by increasing or decreasing the number of students on each relay team.

7) Alter the procedure and have all the students pass through the hoop in the same way: down over the body (head to feet) or up over the body (feet to head).

HOOP ROLL RELAY

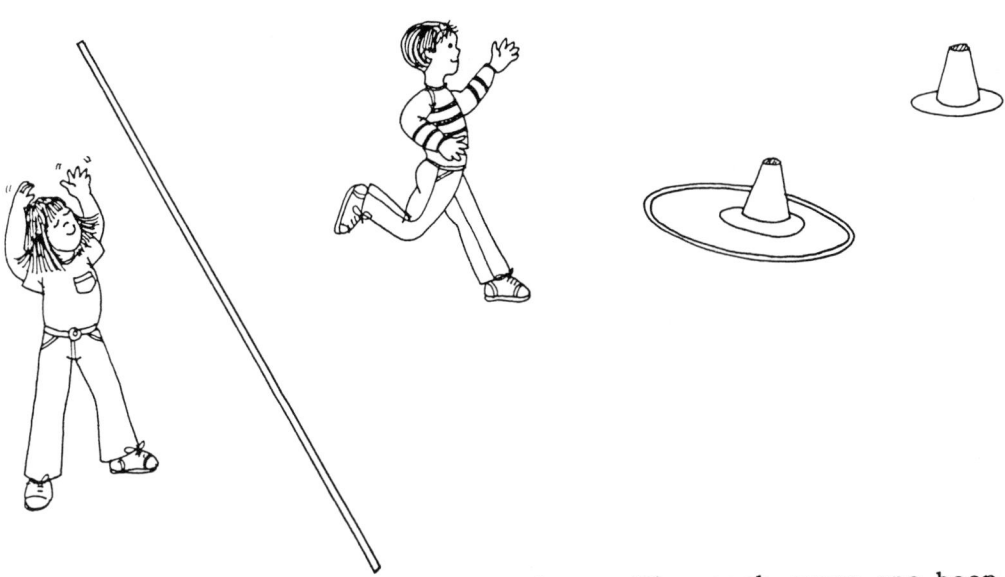

Organize the students into groups of two or three. Give each group one hoop and two large traffic cones or comparable pieces of equipment. Have each group place one cone on a marker twenty feet in front of the foul line and place the second cone on a marker thirty feet in front of the foul line. The two cones are one behind the other and directly in front of the team's designated starting place on the foul line. Set the hoop over the first cone. Instruct the team members to stand one behind the other with the first team member standing on the team's designated starting place on the foul line. On the signal for the relay to begin, the first team member on each team runs to the first cone, picks up the hoop, rolls the hoop to the second cone, sets the hoop over the second cone, runs back to the foul line, and touches the hand of the second team member. The second team member runs to the second cone, picks up the hoop, rolls the hoop to the first cone, sets the hoop over the first cone, runs back to the foul line, and touches the hand of the hand of the third team member or touches the hand of the partner/teammate. This person continues the relay by repeating the procedure performed by the first team member. The two different relay procedures are repeated until the conclusion of the relay race.

ADDITIONAL TEACHING SUGGESTIONS

1) Establish relay teams that are coed and equal in ability levels.

2) Increase or decrease the distances of the traffic cones from the foul line and between each other to meet the ability level and grade level of the students.

3) Instead of stopping the relay race after each team member has taken one turn, continue the relay race for a designated period of time. Ask each student or relay team to count the number of turns taken during the time period, then have each student or relay team share the number at the end of the time period. Even though the activity is competitive, consider lessening the importance of the number of turns taken. Instead, highlight team performance, sportsmanship and fair play, honesty in counting the number of turns and playing by the rules, and individual and team effort displayed throughout the relay race regardless of the outcome.

4) Rotate/change relay team members at the end of each relay race to lessen the competitive feeling and to give all students the opportunity to be on a relay team with other classmates.

5) Discuss the positive aspects of competition.

6) Have the students on each relay team shake hands or display another acceptable form of sportsmanship with members of at least one other relay team at the conclusion of each relay race.

7) Discuss and demonstrate proper and safe touching techniques to allow the next team member to take his/her turn.

8) Make certain the person's hand is touched before he/she begins to take his/her turn. If this student starts to run or crosses the foul line before his/her hand is touched, have the student return to the foul line and repeat the procedure by following the rules of the relay race.

THROUGH THE HOOP RELAY

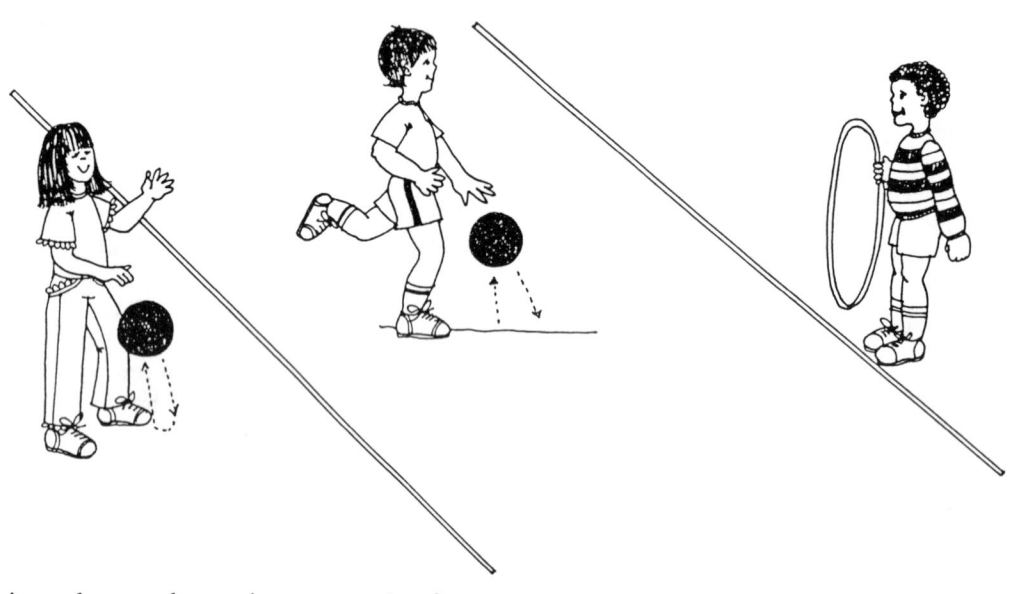

Organize the students into groups of two or three. Give each group one hoop and one or two basketball-size balls determined by the number within the group. Mark a line twenty to thirty feet parallel to the foul line. Instruct the team members to stand one behind the other at a designated starting place on the foul line. The first team member in each line is holding a hoop horizontal to the ground surface. The second team member and, if there are three per group, the third team member are holding balls. On the signal for the relay to begin, the first team member on each team rolls the hoop forward to the marked line. Once at the line, the first team member positions the hoop on the line to be parallel to the foul line. Once the hoop is in the proper position, the second team member hand dribbles his/her ball toward the hoop, passes through the hoop while continuing to dribble the ball, and dribbles the ball to return to the foul line. After the second team member returns to the foul line, the first team member rolls the hoop back to the foul line. If there are two team members per relay team, the members exchange equipment and the relay race progresses with each team member performing the other relay race task. If there are three members per relay team, the first team member gives the hoop to the second team member and exchanges the hoop for the second team member's ball. The first team member moves behind the third team member. The relay race continues with the second team member rolling the hoop forward to the marked line. Once the hoop is in the proper horizontal position on the line, the third team member hand dribbles the ball toward the hoop, passes through the hoop while continuing to dribble the ball, and dribbles the ball to return to the foul line. After the third team member returns to the foul line, the second team member rolls the hoop back to the foul line. If there are two team members per relay team, the members exchange equipment and the relay race continues with each team member repeating the initial relay race task. The switching of relay race tasks continues until the end of the relay race. If there are three members per relay team, the second team member gives the hoop to the third team member and exchanges the hoop for the third team member's ball. The second team member moves behind the first team member. The relay race continues with the third team member rolling the hoop forward to the marked line. Once the hoop is in the proper horizontal position on the line, the first team member hand dribbles the ball toward the hoop, passes through the hoop while continuing to dribble the ball, and dribbles the ball to return to the foul line. After the first team member returns to the foul line, the third team member rolls the hoop back to the foul line. The relay race progresses with the third team member giving the hoop to the first team member and taking the first team member's ball and moving behind the second team member in the line. Once the exchange is made between the first team member and the third team member, the relay race continues with the first team member rolling the hoop toward the foul line. All procedures are repeated until the conclusion of the relay race.

ADDITIONAL TEACHING SUGGESTIONS

1) Establish relay teams that are coed and equal in ability levels.

2) Increase or decrease the distance of the marked line from the foul line to meet the ability level and grade level of the students.

3) Instead of stopping the relay race after each team member has taken one turn, continue the relay race for a designated period of time. Ask each student or relay team to count the number of turns taken during the time period, then have each student or relay team share the number at the end of the time period. Even though the activity is competitive, consider lessening the importance of the number of turns taken. Instead, highlight team performance, sportsmanship and fair play, honesty in counting the number of turns and playing by the rules, and individual and team effort displayed throughout the relay race regardless of the outcome.

4) Rotate/exchange relay team members at the end of each relay race to lessen the competitive feeling and to give all students the opportunity to be on a relay team with fellow classmates.

5) Discuss the positive aspects of competition.

6) Regardless of the number of members on a relay team, have the member(s) with the ball(s) dribble the ball in place during the time the other team member rolls the hoop forward to the marked line and rolls the hoop to return to the foul line.

7) When traveling toward the marked line, have the team member dribble with the dominate hand and have the team member dribble with the opposite hand to return to the foul line.

8) Make certain the team members follow the rules according to the appropriate time to begin to dribble toward the marked line to pass through the hoop and to begin to roll the hoop back to the foul line after the person who has passed through the hoop returns to the foul line. If the rules are not followed, have the student/offender repeat the procedure.

9) Have the students on each relay team shake hands or display another acceptable form of sportsmanship with members of at least one other relay team at the conclusion of each relay race.

BIBLIOGRAPHY

Baltimore County Board of Education. 1982. A GUIDE FOR ELEMENTARY SCHOOL PHYSICAL EDUCATION. Towson, Maryland: Baltimore County Public Schools

Brehm, Madeleine and Tindell, Nancy T. 1983. MOVEMENT WITH A PURPOSE: PERCEPTUAL MOTOR LESSON PLANS FOR YOUNG CHILDREN. West Nyack, New York: Parker Publishing Company, Inc.

Burton, Elsie Carter. 1977. THE NEW PHYSICAL EDUCATION FOR ELEMENTARY SCHOOL CHILDREN. Boston, Massachusetts; Atlanta, Georgia; Dallas, Texas; Geneva, Illinois; Hopewell, New Jersey; Palo Alto, California; and London, England: Houghton Mifflin Company.

Capon, Jack J. 1975. BALL, ROPE, HOOP ACTIVITIES. Carthage, Illinois; Fearon Teacher Aids.

Dauer, Victor P. and Pangrazi, Robert P. (7th ed.). 1983. DYNAMIC PHYSICAL EDUCATION FOR ELEMENTARY SCHOOL CHILDREN. Minneapolis, Minnesota: Burgess Publishing Company.

Davis, R. and Isaacs, L. 1985. ELEMENTARY PHYSICAL EDUCATION: GROWING THROUGH MOVEMENT. Winston-Salem, North Carolina: Hunter Textbooks, Inc.

Lee, A.; Thomas, J.; and Thomas, K. 1989. PHYSICAL EDUCATION FOR CHILDREN: DAILY LESSON PLANS. Champaign, Illinois: Human Kinetics Books.

Lloyd, Marcia L. 1990. ADVENTURES IN CREATIVE MOVEMENT ACTIVITIES: A GUIDE FOR TEACHING. Selangor Darul Eksan, Malaysia: Federal Publications Sdn. Bhd.

Means, C; Taylor, B; and Zanin, E. 1988. ACTIVITIES FOR THE NEW PHYSICAL EDUCATION. Winston-Salem, North Carolina: Hunter Textbooks, Inc.

Short, Kathryn. 1990. PHYSICAL EDUCATION IS MORE THAN KICKBALL. Brea, California: Kathryn Short Productions.

Tillman, Kenneth G. and Toner, Patricia Rizzo. 1983. WHAT ARE WE DOING IN GYM TODAY? West Nyack, New York: Parker Publishing Company, Inc.

Turner, L. and Turner, S. 1982. ELEMENTARY PHYSICAL EDUCATION: MORE THAN JUST GAMES. Palo Alto, California: Peek Publications.

! FREE BROCHURE !

of

SIXTEEN BASIC HOOP SKILLS

Send for a FREE brochure for the Sixteen Basic Hoop Skills Charts
and other products from:

P.E.T.A., Inc.
(Physical Education Teaching Accessories)

Write or Call:

P.E.T.A., Inc.
1023 St. Paul Street
Baltimore, MD 21202

Phone: 1-301-668-9230

! FREE PUBLISHER'S CATALOG !

Send for a FREE catalog of

INNOVATIVE CURRICULUM GUIDEBOOKS AND MATERIALS

in

Movement Education, Special Education and Perceptual-Motor Development

Call Toll-Free: 1-800-524-9091

Or Write:

FRONT ROW EXPERIENCE
540 Discovery Bay Blvd.
Byron, CA 94514-9454